break up with narcissism

HOW TO BREAK FREE
AND **STAY FREE**

Dr. Alina Kastner

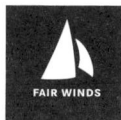

FAIR WINDS

"Narcissist—changing
perception, one deception
at a time."

—Unknown

For each and every one of you
who has been hurt by a narcissist.

contents

introduction

"The narcissist devours people, consumes their output, and casts the empty, writhing shells aside."

—Sam Vaknin

Asking yourself whether you're involved with a narcissist (narc) is a scary place to be. You are probably feeling very alone with some unanswered questions in your head right now. My mission is to help you answer most of those questions. I have been in your shoes many times before and know exactly what it feels like. Even though I dedicated a lot of time to the topic of narcissism, I was not safe from its heartbreak. The pain from these relationships motivated me to learn everything I could about narcissism and help others around the world avoid going through what I did. It pushed me to become a psychotherapist, focus on couples and spousal abuse, and even write a two-hundred-page PhD dissertation on narcissism.

Despite my knowledge of narcissists at the time, I was still deeply hurt by them. If back then I had a simple book that summarized everything I needed know in order to validate my assumptions and escape my abuser sooner, I would have been spared so much heartache and wasted emotional investment.

I'd love you to be able to trace back what has happened with narcissists in your past, understand what is going on with the narcissist in the present, and figure out how to deal with leaving the narcissist going forward. This is exactly what I set out to do with this book. I want to arm you with all the knowledge and emotional preparation you need for this war and give you the necessary wisdom, guidance, and confidence to end it. You can break free and stay free from narcissistic partners forever.

I do not believe in coincidences. There is a solid reason for you to be reading this book right now, and that reason is that you have started your healing journey already, whether you know it or not. This book will help you take off the rose-colored glasses you're still wearing with your narcissist and give you 20/20 vision in order to fully see what is happening and rise in love with yourself.

I will begin by explaining why, in the very beginning, your narcissistic partner may have felt like a little piece of paradise—like your soulmate. Then I will uncover what has truly happened: They lured you into their narcissistic web to manipulate and abuse you. After clarifying why you're experiencing feelings of confusion, hurt, betrayal, and possibly even severe depression, I will guide you through the healing process. This journey includes educating you from a psychological perspective on the dynamics of narcissistic relationships, introducing effective coping mechanisms, and outlining rules for navigating and recovering from such a relationship. This book is designed to help you break free from the toxicity of a narcissistic relationship and get you back in touch with your true self. It's hard to believe, but if you have a little faith in yourself and this process, even if you're not feeling it right now, you will grow stronger through this heart-wrenching experience and your hard work will pay off.

Throughout this book you'll find passages with personal notes and reminders from me to you. These are designed to help you pause, reflect, and engage with the material on a deeper level. This interactive approach isn't just about reading—it's about doing the work for your emotional and spiritual growth. Please ensure you have a journal ready so you can take notes and do these check-in exercises. In the resources section in the back of this book, you will find a self-help journal I made specially for healing after toxic breakups. Take each of these reflection moments seriously, and you'll find the healing process truly begins here.

It all starts with you.

part one

identifying you're in a narcissist's web

chapter 1

unmasking the narcissist

"If it walks like a duck and talks like a duck, it's a duck.
But if it walks like a duck and talks like a swan, it's a narcissist."

—Anonymous

I remember the first time I saw him. His eyes lit up and his smile reached from ear to ear. It was so contagious. He made me feel like I was the only person in the entire restaurant. When he started talking about his love and desire for children within the first five seconds of our date, I was impressed. The first few weeks with him were heaven. He fulfilled all my dream-man, manifest-list bullet points. His work consisted of helping others in hard times, and he always told stories where he saved innocent kids. He was kind to all our friends and showed emotional intelligence like no one ever had. He listened, he cared, he loved. He seemed beautiful inside and out, just like a man made in heaven. He made me breakfast. He was very generous: He listened when others talked, tried to go out of his way to solve my problems, flew in his parents to meet me after just a few weeks, called me gorgeous, made incredible love to me every day and night. He impressed my parents with his intelligence, charm, and talk about soon-to-be-marriage, and all my friends were telling me if they didn't love me so much, they would be jealous. I was so glad to finally meet someone who seemed equally ready: ready to love, ready to give, ready to commit—true romance, intense passion, a loving family life. The kind of love my mom told me doesn't exist. I felt like it would be us against the rest of the world, forever. The whole nine yards. At last, everything I ever wanted. I never could have imagined that this beautiful man would end up putting me through so much emotional torment. He seemed so innocent, so full of love, so ready to give love. But all of that was a deception.

After a few months of a whirlwind romance, I began to realize that no matter how rosy my glasses were, they could no longer hide his true colors. This "perfectly functioning" man was, in reality, a closeted alcoholic with massive control and jealousy issues. Most evenings he would secretly drink to the point of slurring, and when I expressed concern, he'd gaslight me, claiming it was just one glass and starting a fight. He made a scene whenever I met with friends, insisting it was my fault when he got drunk because I "left him home alone," even if it was only for a few hours, and despite my desperate attempts to prove my love and provide constant updates about my whereabouts. He even forbade me from seeing my father, accusing me of loving my father more than him.

If I had to attend an event—birthdays, doctor appointments, or anything else—he would insist on dropping me off and picking me up, ensuring he knew exactly where I was and with whom. He would isolate me nonstop: Over the course of our relationship, we only went out for dinner twice. Every other moment was spent at home because he didn't want anyone, especially any man, to talk to me, touch me (even just a handshake), or look at me. This was his way of maintaining control.

Beyond the explicit rules, there were hundreds of implicit ones. My focus needed to be on him at all times. I wasn't allowed to be "too" successful at work or to be outgoing. I wasn't allowed to cuddle my dog, Amari, more than him or buy furniture for my own apartment with my own money. I wasn't allowed to speak when handypeople came to my house. I wasn't allowed to ask him to contribute to my rent. I was constantly on edge, trying to follow these rules while predicting his next demand so I could behave accordingly. There would be one good day, followed by two bad ones. One good moment of hope, followed by many of grief and despair. The constant anxiety consumed me. Most nights I averaged just three hours of sleep, as he would either keep me up with relentless sexual demands or start arguments that spiraled into five-to-eight-hour monologues from him. He forced me to stay awake and listen until 4 a.m., even though we had to be up by 6:30 a.m. I was so drained and exhausted that people frequently commented on how tired I looked. I saw all the signs.

I thought about leaving him countless times. But as soon as he sensed me withdrawing, he would reel me back in with a dizzying mix of promises to change, horrible threats, and his most convincing tactic: luring me into the dream of having a baby and promising to support me in it. I wasn't strong enough to leave during my first attempts. I stayed to the point where he destroyed my bubbly spirit, every other day leaving me curled up on the floor like an embryo, crying so hard it physically hurt. I didn't understand how I could have fallen for someone like him—again.

I could fill another hundred pages with stories of his behavior, but this book isn't about me—it's about you. I want to spare you the pain I've endured.

Does that sound familiar to you? I bet it does. This is my personal story, but it can happen to anyone. The narcissist will have you believing they are a swan when all they are on the inside is an ugly duckling. It's sometimes very hard to tell who you have in front of you or whom you have fallen for. You need to understand what narcissists are made of. After reading this book, you will.

what is narcissistic personality disorder?

In this day and age, people say "so-and-so is a narcissist" simply because "so-and-so" is acting like a jerk. That's understandable but incorrect. Narcissism is a personality disorder that has very serious mental health implications for anyone involved. It is also a spectrum. Just displaying a narcissistic trait doesn't make someone have a personality disorder. You may encounter narcissists at work or within your family or friends, but this book focuses purely on the experience of having a narcissist as an intimate partner.

I want to give you the only correct way of defining narcissistic personality disorder (NPD), the only real way to find out whether your partner has NPD. To diagnose someone with NPD, mental health professionals use the *Diagnostic and Statistical Manual of Mental Disorders*, 5th edition (DSM-5), the "bible" of psychological disorders.

According to the DSM-5, narcissistic personality disorder consists of nine points:

1. Having a grandiose sense of self-importance

2. Being preoccupied with fantasies of unlimited success and power

3. Believing oneself to be "special" and unique and misunderstood except by other special people

4. Requiring excessive admiration

5. Having an outsize sense of entitlement

6. Being interpersonally exploitative

7. Lacking empathy

8. Being envious

9. Showing arrogant behavior

To be officially diagnosed with NPD, a person must display *at least five out of the nine* behaviors. Only a licensed professional can diagnose someone with NPD, but these nine points can help you determine whether you're dealing with a narcissist.

Just because someone sleeps with you and then ignores you, seems interested and suddenly stops texting, or cheats on you and leaves you and your kids, it does not automatically make them a narcissist. Simply put, acting like a jerk does not directly translate as narcissism; it is simply an expression of narcissistic traits. It's like saying you're depressed when you feel sad—sadness is a trait of depression, but depression involves much more. Likewise, narcissism goes beyond selfishness, arrogance, or a lack of empathy. A true narcissist must meet at least five of the nine criteria listed above to be diagnosed with NPD. Everyone else is simply a person displaying narcissistic traits.

the two types of narcissism

Narcissism can further be differentiated into two categories: the grandiose type ("overt narcissist") and the vulnerable type ("covert narcissist").

Most people know about *grandiose narcissists*. The grandiose narcissist is defined by their fearless, confident, and approach-oriented behavior. They have a strong desire to dominate their partner, which they exert by avoiding deep emotional attachments to them. To gain control and power over their partner, they induce feelings of inferiority by making them feel fearful, jealous, and anxious through spite, antagonism, and hostility. This behavior always keeps you on your toes. While the grandiose type may appear to have decent self-esteem, they are actually fragile. They desperately need to maintain their pretentious self-image and need for admiration and attention. At first they charm their way into your heart with their seeming kindness and magnetic charisma. They seem to exert a gravitational pull on you. Not only will they fool you but your friends and family are highly likely to fall for their show as well. They seem to be in a relationship all the time, but they rarely have long-lasting ones. After a while of being around them, you will find that they are incredibly self-absorbed and constantly need to be in the spotlight.

The *vulnerable narcissist* seems neurotic, fearful, and shy. Unlike the grandiose narcissist, the vulnerable narcissist comes across as reserved at first as they try to avoid tension and conflict. Because they lack self-esteem and oscillate between feelings of superiority and inferiority, it is harder to identify them as dangerous. To gain control and power over their intimate partner, they will play the victim to get their partner's sympathy and attention. They use passive-aggressive behavior to show their anger and frustration, leaving their partner feeling guilty. This in turn allows them to maintain their facade of innocence for a longer time. Just like the grandiose narc, they are highly sensitive to criticism; they won't allow it. They will guilt-trip you into feeling sorry for them and through this make you fulfill their wishes, which often ends with you neglecting your own needs and being exploited.

CHECK-IN

I'm sure you can think of several situations when the "spotlight" should have been on you, but seconds later it was back on them. Or a situation where you were made to feel guilty, jealous, or anxious because of their behavior. Write these situations down in your journal so you don't forget about all these painful instances, and let your friends remind you if you don't remember the pain these situations inflicted on you.

Both grandiose and vulnerable narcissists hide their insecurities behind their mask of confidence. Once you start questioning this mask, you will often find them twisting the truth, causing you to doubt your judgment or memory of what just happened. You will be blamed for whatever it is that *they* did, which will lead you to question your sanity. This is what is called gaslighting. The impact of being gaslit for too long often leads to mental health issues, self-doubt, complete devastation, and occasionally homicide or suicide.

> **WARNING**
>
> If you are feeling suicidal in any way, no self-help book in the world can provide you with enough support. Please lay down this book and immediately reach out to a mental health professional or suicide hotline, and let your family and friends know that you are not okay. It is not in your head; research confirms that there is an overlap between grandiose narcissism and psychopathy, and psychopaths will always aim to destroy you completely.

The narc might gaslight you into believing that their behavior is all your fault, that you drive them to act the way they do. Nothing could be further from the truth. You did not "cause" their problems: Their childhood did.

what causes NPD?

Children who receive "adequate" love, nurture, and care from their parent or primary caregiver before the age of three learn ways to regulate their emotions appropriately. For instance, with "adequate" parents, when a child is angry due to not getting what they want, the child can voice that anger, feel it, and then self-regulate to acceptance. The child is given a safe and secure space from their parents to be allowed to feel their uncomfortable emotion (such as anger) and not get punished for it. These parents will help the child deal with difficult emotions until the child can manage their feelings on their own.

This does not mean that a child is always allowed to act however they want. Parents who let their child act however they want foster narcissism by teaching and tolerating entitlement. A part of healthy parenting simply means that children are allowed to experience their range of emotions and still be loved unconditionally. When children are allowed to feel all types of feelings, learn social norms for dealing with them, understand the rules and regulations regarding their behavior, and yet still feel safe while experiencing difficult emotions, they develop healthy self-esteem, also known as "healthy narcissism." Healthy narcissism is a universal aspect of child development cultivated by imitating, also known as *mirroring*, the parents' confidence and self-esteem. Children implicitly learn rules of behavior through mirroring. Only if parents are "adequately healthy" will the child find healthy confidence and self-esteem by mirroring them.

Mirroring goes both ways. Parents can also mirror the child by imitating and reflecting back their behaviors, attitudes, and emotional states. For example, when a baby is smiling, an attentive parent will smile back at them, making them feel seen and validated. The parent is mirroring the child's smile, helping them feel understood and connected. When a child witnesses the parent coping with a negative feeling such as disappointment or frustration in a healthy manner, they learn that emotions come and go and can be managed. This teaches them not to be overwhelmed by their internal state.

Since every child wants to be like their parents, the child will always follow their parents' lead, also known as idealization. Idealization is the child's certainty that their parents are perfect. In the beginning, every child experiences this phenomenon. Children view their parents as all-powerful, omnipresent, perfect beings in order to feel safe, secure, and protected. This increases the trust bond between children and their parents, which is the base for role modeling. Through this bond, children learn to copy their parents' behaviors and values. This shapes the child's sense of self and their understanding of the world.

Mirroring and idealization with healthy parents lead to self-confident children. Self-confident children are much more able to enjoy social activities such as sports and form new friendships. These children are respectful of boundaries because they understand their importance and will thus adapt better to circumstances around them while also being able to state their own boundaries in an emotionally intelligent way. Both mirroring and idealization phases gradually fade and are exchanged with more realistic truths and views. Children later come to understand that nobody is perfect; their parents have flaws, and that is okay. They learn to regulate their expectations toward themselves and others—family, friends, partners. They know that being human means that everyone—including themselves!—has flaws, and yet they can still authentically love and maintain genuine relationships.

On the other hand, when parents neglect the child, the child starts to develop coping mechanisms to survive these harsh conditions. They learn very early on how to fine-tune their antenna in order to read people around them, so they in turn get what they need to survive, such as food, affection, attention. This is subconscious and not "bad" in babies—it is a pure survival mechanism.

Frederick II, the king of Sicily, conducted a diabolic experiment in the thirteenth century where he took babies from their mothers at birth and placed them in nurses' care. He was trying to find out what language they would speak if no one spoke to them. He imposed two rules: The nurses weren't allowed to talk to or hold the babies. To his surprise, the babies all died. Tragically, this experiment proves that babies who aren't "loved"—by receiving cuddles, warmth, and proper interaction—literally die, even if they are fed and maintained hygienically.

While this experiment proves that babies who receive no love die, we now can derive that babies who receive inadequate love (some talking, some holding, some feedings, some hygiene) survive but carry a deficiency within them forever—a deficiency so deep that it's irreparable. So, if these babies are not "treated right," and if circumstances don't change within the first three years of their lives, this can lead to continuous unhealthy coping behaviors during later years and through adulthood. They stay stuck in the stage of baby survival, always ensuring they get what they need. They use their antennae to read what their partner needs, giving it to them for the time being (i.e., love-bombing), not with heartfelt intention but as a necessity to get something back for themselves—to feel loved and admired. This is what a narcissist does, and they won't ever change without professional help. Their wound is too deep. A narcissist feels they would die without this validation, and this would have been true for them as a baby.

I share this not to make you feel sorry for them but rather to let you know how their lack developed and that it sits so deep that you can't undo it. You cannot go back in time and heal this wound for them; it will stay with them forever unless they do the work. No amount of love in the present will make up for the missing love from their past.

Alternatively, when children are "overnourished" with excessive praise or are made to feel that their problems are exceptional and that they are superspecial, they can develop a sense of entitlement, believing they have the right to act in morally questionable ways or hurt others while disregarding social norms. Children naturally think they are the center of the world, and part of growing up is learning that they are not. However, if the parent has not taught them how to manage their naturally selfish impulses, they will not move on to the phase where they develop a realistic view about the world. They remain stuck in the developmental stage of a child and hold unrealistic expectations of perfection—the beginning of what could end up as narcissism. They want to think they are flawless, and they expect others to be as well. Since this unrealistic expectation cannot be met, they bounce back and forth between idealizing (everything is perfect) and devaluing (oh no, everything is not perfect, and I hate everyone for it). Their inflated sense of self-importance often alternates with deep feelings of unworthiness when they cannot maintain their "special" status, leading to a fragile and unstable sense of self.

Parents who neglect or overly idealize their child typically demonstrate a lack of empathy, failing to understand and respond properly to the child's age-appropriate needs. This lack of sufficient love and appropriate care leads to impaired emotional functioning and constant intense feelings of fear, abandonment, and self-doubt. Thus, this child grows up to be a narcissistic individual who tries their whole life to have their childlike needs met by others, specifically by their intimate partner. Due to the void left by their parents, they expect their partner to serve as a substitute to fill this void.

CHECK-IN

While intimately involved with a narcissist, you may feel like it is your sole responsibility to fill this void for them. You cannot save them. This is an old wound that they carry. Write down some moments where you felt responsible for their void and they made you feel guilty for not fulfilling your "duty" to perfection. Was there something more you felt you had to do to be enough and deserving of their love?

Narcissists are exploitative and, more often than not, treat their partner as an object of supply for them, not as a human being. They often experience massive mood swings that stir up lots of trouble in intimate relationships. Due to their preoccupation with fantasies of power, larger-than-life success or beauty, the ideal family, and perfect love, narcissists even become envious of their intimate partner and, of course, others they perceive as "having more than them" or "having it all." Their insecurity may manifest as an empty well. With a narcissist, you keep trying to fill their empty well with everything you have, but it will never suffice. This is why you can never win with a narcissist, even if you try to set yourself on fire to keep them warm. Instead, giving them so much of you will take a huge emotional toll on you.

your emotional toll

How much of an emotional toll is your relationship costing you? You can use the following checklist to find out. If more than five of these points apply, you are in an abusive relationship with a narcissist:

1. As much as my partner compliments me, I still feel judged at times.
2. I am afraid that if I do something wrong, my partner will cause a huge scene or threaten to leave me.
3. I am constantly being blamed for my partner's mistakes or problems.
4. I am constantly confused about how they feel about me; I never feel consistently safe or loved.
5. I cannot share my problems with others because my partner has made me feel as though it is wrong to share our problems, often calling me dramatic or making me feel very guilty, as if I'm trying to ruin our relationship.
6. I feel as though I am being made to doubt my judgments, memories, and sanity (also known as gaslighting).
7. I feel as though my feelings are not taken seriously.
8. I feel like I need to walk on eggshells to avoid upsetting my partner.
9. I have begun to believe my partner's criticisms of me; maybe it is all my fault.
10. I never know what part of them I am going to encounter each day.
11. I start to question my own truth and reality.
12. None of our friends and family ever sees the dark side of them.

13. One minute I feel loved and appreciated, then the next minute I am receiving the silent treatment or have an angry partner at home.

14. The relationship often feels one-sided.

15. There are ridiculous amounts of fighting, and it never seems to be constructive.

Does any of this sound familiar? You've likely experienced most of the above. You need to know that their need for narcissistic supply is what's wearing down your mental health and ruining your relationship. It's not your lack of ability or worth, it's not your fault, and there is nothing you can do about it except not follow their rules. Which leads me to the Ten Commandments of Narcissistic Supply.

the ten commandments of narcissistic supply

It is perfectly natural for everyone to want the "supplies" of feeling admired, loved, and respected to be fulfilled every now and then in order to live a happy life full of self-worth. Sometimes we do things in our favor to the detriment of someone else: We act selfishly, want to control things, or manipulate others. Still, a healthy person is able to reflect and engage in self-questioning through their internal system of checks and balances. When we realize we are taking more than we are giving, we will adjust our behaviors, apologize, feel remorse, and grow. All of this is perfectly human.

The key difference with the narcissist is their intent and the intensity of their needs. They have an extreme and relentless need for all these supply points to be constantly fulfilled at the highest level, especially by you. They never question the reciprocity in the relationship, whether the give-and-take is balanced or fair. They expect full-fledged dedication to their needs and don't plan on returning the favor unless it is part of their calculated strategy to get something for themselves. *A narcissist never gives without expecting to get.* If you do not fulfill all the narcissist's supply needs at all times, you will start to see rapid shifts in their behavior, as their charade begins to crumble.

The following "Ten Commandments of Narcissistic Supply" show how these traits can manifest in your everyday life. If more than half apply to your situation, you know for certain that your partner is a narcissist.

1. grandiosity:

"You Shall Have No Other Gods Before Me!"

a. Your partner has an exaggerated sense of self-importance and is always disproportionately inflating their value:

> *"My boss praised me today because . . ."*
> *"I gave so much of me to my crazy bipolar ex . . ."*
> *"I had to walk our dog today even though it was so hot, and I actually had so much work to catch up on . . ."*

b. Your partner always thinks they are superior and only likes to associate with equally "special" people:

> *"I think so-and-so isn't as religious as we are . . ."*
> *"I don't want to associate with . . ."*
> *"I think so-and-so is morally questionable—I mean, they left their partner and two kids . . ."*

2. admiration:

"You Shall Not Covet Anyone Like You Do Me!"

a. Your partner constantly seeks excessive admiration and attention—especially from you but also from everyone else:

> *"I am the best at my job. Everyone else is useless . . ."*
> *"I put up those shelves so fast, I bet no one else could have done it that fast!"*

Afterward, they expect you to praise them for their accomplishment like a little child seeking approval.

b. Your partner requires constant validation and praise from you and others to feel important. For example, if your partner does not receive praise from you after a few days, you will start to feel it because they will start putting you down. If others begin to praise you instead of them, it is reason enough for them to freak out or cause a scene, calling you conceited or arrogant.

3. entitlement:

"Honor Your Narcissist!"

a. Your partner has unreasonable expectations of especially favorable treatment from everyone. For example, your partner expects you to revolve your schedule around them at all costs, as they are unwilling to compromise, even if they have much less on their plate than you do. They force vacations on you that you can't afford or that fall below your expectations. They prefer to invite their friends to gatherings rather than yours or they don't invite you to their gatherings at all. They make sure they hijack every one of your special events in order to steal your happiness about them (holiday gatherings, weddings, your birthday). They prefer to always do things for themselves rather than for you. They expect you to emotionally support them through their roller coaster of needs while constantly ignoring your needs.

b. Your partner believes they deserve more—appreciation, love, respect, admiration—than anyone else and expects automatic compliance with their expectations from you. For example, your partner tends to state their needs and desires as highly important and expects you to always cater to them, because their needs always take precedence over yours. At the same time, they will complain that all they do is cater to your needs. This also applies to decisions about social events or finances.

c. Your partner is so intensely preoccupied with their own problems and interests to the point it becomes infuriating. For example, when something comes up in your life that you need to prioritize, they will refuse to acknowledge it and continue their victim play. They will constantly talk about how difficult their life is, all the things they need to do, how they are exhausted. They will complain about always being a helper and how much they give up for others. They will make it a point how they are being exploited at work. Or they will kick aside the victim mask and role-play their importance by continuously putting their interests before the interests of your partnership and you. They will go work out at the most inopportune times, perhaps when you need them at home to help with something or during the middle of an important conversation. When you mention this to them, they will say you are jealous that they take better care of themselves and you should simply do the same. During this whole time, your partner obviously shows little or no concern for your needs.

4. exploitative behavior:

"You Shall Not Question Me!"

a. Your partner takes advantage of you and anyone around them in order to get what they want. This often involves you helping them fulfill their projects while not getting your own done, helping them get promoted but ignoring and not supporting your work life, or using you to take care of their kids and always complaining how horrible you are at it.

b. Your partner uses manipulation or deceit to get what they want. This happens very dangerously in financial situations where your partner will ask you to co-sign something without making clear to you what the contract entails. It can also mean hijacking beautiful moments, like pretending to be sick when you're out with friends or starting a fight before a holiday dinner with your family. They will start fights with you before social gatherings and then pretend like nothing happened as soon as you arrive; they will act happy and kind in public around others, while you are still upset and trying to shake off what just happened. They do this to be seen as the "good one" in front of your family and friends and to paint you as the "crazy one" who is always in a bad mood, further isolating you. Another common exploitative behavior is accusing you of being overly jealous or paranoid while they're cheating. Or they'll induce jealousy in you, leading you to doubt your own perceptions and become weaker.

5. lack of empathy:

"You Shall Not Expect Compassion from Me!"

a. Your partner is unwilling to recognize or identify with your feelings and needs. For example, they might have pretended to be overly understanding or empathetic in the beginning, but when push comes to shove, they'll make very clear that actually they don't care. They can leave you unanswered or on "read" for hours and seemingly not have an issue when there is an elephant in the room. They ignore you and it doesn't seem to faze them—ever. They show little to no interest in your emotions or experiences when they don't want to. It is scary how unimpressed they can be when you break down in front of them, beg, or cry. They might just tell you to "stop being dramatic" or "get over yourself, this is pathetic," when all you need is a hug or reassurance.

6. envious behavior:

"You Shall Not Outshine Me!"

a. Your partner often feels envious of you or believes that you are envious of them. For instance, you will find your narcissistic partner competing with you over the most ridiculous things—work accomplishments, who does a chore better, who is the better parent, who is fitter at the gym. *They don't seem to want to understand that partners should complement each other, not compete with one another.*

b. Your partner reacts negatively to your successes or happiness. When good things are happening for you, they seem to be out to destroy your luck or make you feel guilty or undeserving of it. When you reach a milestone for yourself, they are not supportive or proud but react aggressively in one way or another. Their envy is so appalling that you find yourself not sharing good things that happen to you out of fear of their negative reaction.

7. arrogant attitude:

"You Shall Not Challenge My Superiority!"

a. Your partner constantly displays arrogant behaviors or attitudes, such as being dismissive and rolling their eyes at you, interrupting you, or putting you down. They also love to belittle anything about you, whether that's personality traits, achievements, intelligence, or looks—whatever will hit you the hardest. They know your insecurities and will use every one of them against you by constantly criticizing you. For example, if you do not get along with your mother, they will throw it in your face and say things like, "No wonder your mother doesn't talk to you anymore. Now I understand her." Everything you have ever shared with them in confidence, they will unpack and throw it at you in the most hurtful ways.

b. Your partner acts superior to you by patronizing you for being weak or dumb. They also love to publicly humiliate you, whether that is in front of friends or family, while showing off any chance they can. This often starts as a "joke" and gets worse and even more hurtful with time.

8. control and manipulation:

"You Shall Do as I Say without Question!"

a. Your partner constantly controls and manipulates your actions and decisions. The control and manipulation start subtly. At first they will ask, but then they will start to demand or insist. It can begin with requests such as asking you to not wear something, to not meet a particular person because that person makes them uncomfortable, or to change the way you act when you're in public. These little changes sneak up on you, and you find yourself feeling a bit off but trying to incorporate their wishes into your daily routine. After a while it gets more serious: They will drop you off and pick you up from work or meetings with friends or colleagues, pretending to be sweet but aiming to control you. They will focus all their attention on what you are doing—for example, texting "too much" with friends or still being Instagram friends with a person they don't approve of—which steers attention away from what *they* are doing—blatantly lying; secretly texting or cheating, often with their ex. They will use guilt, intimidation, or other tactics to manipulate you and shape you into the person they want you to be, all without you realizing it.

b. Instead of addressing issues, your partner will triangulate you by comparing you to someone else—who, according to them, is always better than you. One classic act of triangulation is when your partner compares you to their ex, not by criticizing the ex but by putting them on a pedestal. For example, your partner will tell you how unbelievably good their ex is with kids—implying that you are not as good without actually saying it. If you ask them about it, they will call you paranoid and say they never said or meant that. But your gut knows better, even if you don't want to believe it. This is psychological warfare. It leaves you feeling insecure, wondering why they broke up with their ex in the first place and whether they want to go back to them. Their intent is to make you worry so that you adhere to their often intense and insane demands out of fear that they might leave you (as their perfect ex is waiting for them with open arms—and of course wants them back so badly). They will do this by saying things like, "My ex was never jealous of others when I am out"—the intention being to make you hold back from voicing your worries or feelings when a gut instinct is telling you otherwise.

9. the flawless one:

"You Shall Not Bear False Witness against Me!"

a. Your partner does not react well to criticism or critique. They constantly react negatively or aggressively to even perceived criticism at all times. They seem to *want* to understand everything the wrong way or to sabotage the peace between the two of you. (They do.) When you confront them with something, they become defensive, angry, or dismissive; they never own their mistakes or take accountability or responsibility for their behavior. Instead, they'll turn it around on you.

b. Your partner will not take responsibility or accountability for their actions. They have a history of troubled relationships and constantly blame their exes for the failed relationships, not taking an ounce of responsibility. Anyone can have a series of "failed" relationships, but the key thing here is accountability and what you say about your ex. If all their exes were "crazy, bipolar, borderline," this is a massive red flag. We all might have one or two "crazy" exes in our lives, but surely not all of them were "crazy."

10. inconsistent behavior:

"You Shall Not Expect Consistency but Be Happy with My Breadcrumbs!"

a. Your partner displays inconsistent behavior, being loving and sweet one moment and extremely cruel the next. This might be the most devastating of all tactics because it is so unbearable, so unpredictable. It is "casually cruel," as Taylor Swift would say, and it throws off the best of us. This hot-and-cold pattern is detrimental to your health. It causes you to experience heartache, emotional and physical exhaustion, heightened anxiety, and decreased self-efficacy. This is part of the grand scheme of gaslighting, as it truly makes you question your ability to comprehend reality.

b. The sad truth is, if your partner displays several of these characteristics, they may be a narcissist. There is absolutely nothing you can do to "win" this fight and be happy with them. They will not change, no matter how many empty apologies they give (if they even bother to apologize). They don't want to change, even if they swear they will. Now is the time to realize what is happening *and take responsibility for your own happiness.*

> ### CHECK-IN
>
> *Take a few minutes of quiet time during your day and reflect on which of these commandments your partner enforces. Maybe you can even think of things not listed here. Then ask yourself, "How much longer am I willing to tolerate this one-sided, awful treatment?" Write the question in your journal and write your answer so you can come back to it later.*

If you think that getting into this relationship is all your fault, it's not. It might surprise you to know that the narcissist picked you for some very specific reasons.

why did the narcissist pick me?

You might be asking yourself why the narcissist picked you. We often hear that you must be "broken" or "unhealthy" to fall for a con artist like a narcissist. The most common belief is that the narcissist picks weak people—people with low self-esteem who are easy to handle. As a therapist with over a decade of experience counseling clients in abusive relationships, and as a successful and independent woman who has been picked by narcs over and over, I have learned that often the opposite is true. I've found that narcissists tend to choose prey they consider impressive to show off and easy to consume. What do I mean by that? You're great to show off if one or more of the following is true:

- You're beautiful and elevate them with your looks.
- You can entertain a crowd.
- You're witty, self-sufficient, successful, smart, and accomplished.

Narcissists usually seek these types of strong, independent, successful, and often very beautiful partners because they upgrade the narcissist's appearance. In the beginning they will love you for these qualities; later they will hate you for them! They love choosing prey with a good career, as that will positively reflect on them. But later they will blame you for it and compete with you on this front. Ideally you are accomplished and self-sufficient, which makes them have to put in less financial effort or, in many cases, piggyback off of you financially.

Do not feel ashamed for falling for a narcissist. No one is immune to them, not even specialized professionals in the field (wink-wink). Narcissists are drawn to people who are strong-willed and have special talents or characteristics they admire in order to boost their ego. A strong partner makes them feel their own worth is of higher value.

chapter 2

recognizing narcissistic abuse

"Nobody can be kinder than the narcissist while you react to life on his terms."

—Elizabeth Bowen

A narcissist is unbeatable at leaving a good first impression. Their outgoing, self-assured personality attracts you to them like a moth to a light. A narcissist tends to behave in an expressive, self-confident manner and place high importance on grooming themselves and staying physically attractive. Their alluring charm mixed with self-composure gives them an advantage over introverts: mating success. In other words, narcissists are successful in short-term mating because they manage to fascinate their targets right from the start.

why you fell for the narcissist

In the beginning, a narcissist makes you believe you've found your absolute soulmate, your one-and-only, your person. They raise you up and put you on a pedestal until you get used to the intensity of nonstop love-bombing, which usually happens within a few days. Love-bombing is when the narcissist excessively showers you with praise and flattery. They might constantly text and call you, flood you with compliments and affection, talk about marriage early on, and rush to introduce you to their family. They may claim they've never felt this way before, book vacations, plan your future together, and make grand gestures. You'll be frequently bombarded with flowers, gifts, and public displays of affection, spending nonstop time together. They will also physically spoil you: constantly reaching for your hand, hugging you, kissing you, and looking at you with love-filled eyes. They might even talk about having children and starting a family, all designed to make you feel like the most special person in the world. It feels like you are living your very own fairy tale.

This is why you fell for the narcissist.

But all this seemingly unconditional love has an agenda—an agenda that you don't know about yet. They are secretly scheming to get you hooked on their overly loving ways, words, gestures, and actions, causing you to invest more in the relationship than you normally would at such an early stage. You will give them all of yourself and let your guard down quickly, thinking you have found "the one."

During this phase of the relationship, you actively start making future plans together. News flash—your narc will not follow through with these plans! These shared visions of the future give you a false sense of safety and being truly seen. You feel like you have finally found a home in someone. If you didn't receive proper support from your family of origin, this kind of romance feels like the first time you have experienced belonging and, with that, true peace. The narcissist makes you feel like you've found what you've been subconsciously searching for your whole life. You no longer have to look for anyone else or face life alone.

Your soul is finally calm, and this makes you incredibly grateful and committed to your lover. You love this person with everything you have and everything you are. You give the narcissist all of you, and *they know it*. This is exactly where the plot twist creeps in and things begin to unravel. Once the narc has you in their pocket, they will rip all the wonderful "love" away from under your feet and drop you lower than you've ever been before, leaving you completely blindsided.

That is exactly what narcissists do.
They tricked you.
They got you.
And now they can abuse you.

the three types of narcissistic abuse

Narcissistic abuse in intimate relationships has different facets: sexual abuse (coercion, unwanted touching, rape), physical abuse (hitting, battering), and psychological or emotional abuse (the five cycles of narcissistic abuse). All three forms of abuse are excruciating and often intertwined. For example, there is no battering without emotional abuse attached to it. Let's look at each type in more detail, starting with sexual abuse.

1. sexual abuse

You may be exposed to sexual abuse in your relationship with a narcissist. Sexual abuse is not only rape. Sexual abuse within a romantic relationship can start off with "little" things, such as repeatedly pressuring you into sexual acts ("If you love me, you will do this! Everyone else does it!"), ignoring your sexual boundaries, or continuing sexual acts after you have asked them to stop. These acts will increase in intensity and can range from verbally pressuring you into submitting to unwanted kisses to physically forcing intercourse.

If sexual abuse is part of your experience, you are more likely to suffer from stress symptoms compared to a narcissistic relationship that does not include sexual abuse, as these relationships tend to be more brutal overall. Sexual violence, including marital or relationship rape, can instill in victims fear, anxiety, and often severe depression. This often leads to long-term psychological trauma such as post-traumatic stress disorder (PTSD) or complex post-traumatic stress disorder (C-PTSD), which I will describe in more detail later.

The violation that stems from sexual abuse strips you of your dignity and sense of self, leaving you feeling powerless and disconnected from yourself. It can destroy your confidence and even lead to sexual dysfunction. This compounded abuse exponentially increases the toxic dynamics of the relationship, leaving you in a state of constant emotional and psychological turmoil, making it even more impossible to break free.

2. physical abuse

Physical abuse, also known as domestic violence, has a significant impact on your mental health, and recovery can be a long, hard road. This type of abuse leaves both obvious and hidden scars. It's no secret that many physically abused partners hide their circumstances from the outside world by covering up their beatings and bruises. They begin to lie in order to "keep the peace" and often don't even notice when they start to lose their own voice by trying to protect their abuser. Once this happens, survivors often don't realize that they are so deeply in the physical-abuse cycle, trying not to get beat up, that they can't see the forest from the trees and thus forget that there is a possibility of a peaceful life without violence out there. Often they are so consumed with trying to prevent the next outburst that they have no capacity left to strategize how to get out of their situation. They simply try to prevent more beatings rather than leave.

If you are experiencing physical abuse, you will feel drained in all aspects: physically, spiritually, emotionally, and psychologically. It is even common to experience decreased cognitive ability, increased memory loss, and PTSD. Confusion, forgetfulness, and fogginess set in. You may feel burned-out, exhausted, and unable to sleep. Many survivors also develop dependency issues, whether that is alcohol, over-the-counter drug abuse, or narcotics, often leading to more problems. No matter what, after experiencing physical abuse, trauma is inevitable.

3. psychological abuse

Undeniably, sexual and physical abuse put you in grave danger. Yet still, many survivors report that *psychological abuse is the hardest to handle*. This may be because psychological abuse seems invisible. Psychological abuse is behavior that aims to cause emotional or mental harm. It does not leave any physical proof or detectable damage on your body. Rather, it leaves invisible damage to your psyche and soul.

This invisibility to the outside world can make you feel like you can never properly recover from what happened because you can't pinpoint it. You may feel like no one believes you when you describe the torture as it seems so abstract that it is almost impossible to grasp if you haven't been there yourself. Without outside support, there is no one to reflect the reality that you are in a toxic relationship and no one to tell you that it is not your fault. As a result, this sense of being alone, the isolation, causes your thoughts to turn inward and you begin to believe you are to blame for the situation.

What makes psychological abuse so destructive is how it affects you on a deeper, emotional level. In psychological abuse, patterns of control, intimidation, and manipulation cause your emotional boundaries to be crossed constantly, exploiting the trust you once had in yourself, your decision-making, and the outside world. This decreases your perceived independence, empowerment, and resilience, leading you to feel worthless, as if you've lost your identity. The more these boundary violations happen, the more you lose your sense of self and the more your abuser grows in power. The constant criticism of your appearance, intelligence, ability, and very essence of your being begins to take a heavy toll. You may experience insomnia or oversleeping, eating disorders (lack of appetite or overeating), poor personal hygiene, depression, and anxiety, among other symptoms. Ongoing abuse can destroy all your plans and goals in life, your ideals and hopes.

the abuse cycle

Now you know why you fell for the narcissist. But why have you remained in the relationship? Why can't you seem to leave? It's actually very simple: Their cycling between charm and abuse has created a feedback loop in your brain. Let's explore what I mean by this.

Abuse comes in different shapes and sizes, but what is always present during narcissistic abuse is the alternating five-phase cycle. In her book *Becoming the Narcissist's Nightmare*, Shahida Arabi explains the five specific phases of the narcissistic abuse cycle:

1. Idealization
2. Devaluation/De-idealization
3. Discard
4. Destroy
5. Hoover

These phases are designed to control you and exploit you to maintain emotional control over you *at all times*. It is important to understand these phases in order to recognize the extremely harmful dynamics that these abusive relationships consist of. The abuse cycle most often leads to serious psychological consequences and can happen either overtly (evident and apparent to others) or covertly (kept concealed between the narcissist and you, their victim). It leaves psychological, spiritual, and emotional scars that sometimes take a lifetime to heal.

It is my mission to ensure that this will not be you.

1. idealization

In this phase, the narcissist blinds you with love and attention. This phase is the so-called honeymoon phase, and it feels Hollywood amazing. The narcissist tries to make you dependent on them as they mirror your biggest hopes, fantasies, and romantic dreams. Since they are skilled manipulators, they create an incredible love story, learn your love language, and tell you exactly what you want to hear. In this phase, sex is usually incredible as they tune in to your longings, desires, and wishes. Their initial chivalry masks their cruelty. This phase is usually pure happiness for both the victim and the narcissist, making you feel absolutely perfect, which bolsters the narcissist's self-esteem. You basically become addicted to their love.

Kate's Story

"When I first met him, it felt as if the world had finally aligned in my favor. He was everything I had ever dreamed of—charming, attentive, and seemingly perfect. He knew exactly how to make me feel loved and cherished with surprise dates, heartfelt compliments, and promises of a future that seemed too good to be true."

During the idealization phase, you do nothing but make love, plan your future together, talk about children, and have deep, meaningful conversations about life, love, and inner values. There is an endless stream of smiles and laughter, leaving your cheeks sore. The narcissist perfectly presents all the romantic gestures that go along with this behavior. You are nonstop engaged in answering messages from your lover, and they are bombarding you with sweet phone calls, showering you with compliments, posting you all over their social media, and making you feel like you are their "one-in-a-billion prince/princess." You feel you have found your anchor in life; you feel validated, a sense of belonging, cared for, and no longer lonely. All this love showering gets you used to laser-focused attention and daily praise, as well as the typically stunning sex life filled with the exact right mix of tenderness and aggression. At this stage, victims are often bragging to friends about the intense teared-up eye contact you have while making love to each other.

Emma's Story

"He made me feel as though he had finally found the love of his life in me. With tears of emotion, at fifty-six years old, he repeatedly told me that he now understood what love was and why people get married. He promised to love my children as his own and even imagined caring for me in my old age. He was constantly writing letters, drawing pictures, and making crafts—once, he decorated my bed with red paper hearts he had cut out himself, each labeled with an adjective he thought described me (pretty, funny, sexy, intelligent, warmhearted, and so on). He sent me countless WhatsApp messages every day, making me feel like an absolute priority in his life. For the first time, I felt truly seen and appreciated, and I thought, 'This must be true love!'"

As far as hobbies are concerned, the narcissist also mirrors your favorite interests and exploits your viewpoints on life. This makes you feel even more validated, as though you have found a soulmate in the other person—someone special who loves to share their entire world. You start emotionally depending on all the praise from the narcissist and the beautiful time spent together. This fusion creates a biochemical dependence on the narcissist, called a trauma bond, which will be described later in more detail.

CHECK-IN

Unfortunately, indications or alarm signals of how to foresee any sort of abuse are difficult to differentiate from feelings of passionately falling in love. The key to help you differentiate between passionately falling in love and being love-bombed is by observing your partner's consistency over time. A good benchmark is around six months, when things typically begin to change. In your journal, write down the ways they love-bombed you in the beginning of the relationship and the ways they are treating you now.

Even the most perfectly engineered idealization phase fails to be flawless. There is always one slip of the tongue, one rough joke, one remark early on that could raise doubt or at least awareness. A narcissist tests boundaries very early on, trying to see how far they can go with you. *The trick is to see it right away.* It is rare for victims to realize that a game is being played and the extent of the masquerade. It is very difficult to not cling onto the happy fairy tale playing out in front of your eyes and equally difficult to start exploring the red flags. Since this first phase is so intensely beautiful, so lovely, so nourishing for you, it's almost impossible to consider leaving. Even if you are aware that you could be walking into a narcissistic trap, hope dies last. You desperately long to be that one special person they change for, and so you ignore the sneak peeks of the red flags through their sparkly show.

A few lucky individuals see through the trap and leave the relationship right away. Unfortunately most continue investing their emotions and love, unable to look at the red flags, only to move on to the next phase of an intimate relationship with a narcissist—a more unpleasant one.

Monica's Story

"All seemed perfect, even if she frequently told me about other girls who flirted with her and who wanted to have sex with her. I felt secure at that time, so I didn't notice that first alarm in my mind until it became a constant companion."

2. devaluation/de-idealization

The second phase of dating a narcissist is the devaluation or de-idealization phase, which is exactly what it sounds like. The narc takes away all the praise and idealization they gave you in the first phase and begins to devalue you. Initially this process starts slowly, but then it accelerates, leaving you internally destroyed and questioning what has happened, unable to make sense of it. The positive moments become rarer, while the negative aspects steadily grow until they dominate the relationship. In the process of devaluing you, a narcissist is very manipulative. They manage to pick on your weaknesses and traumas while diminishing your strengths, accomplishments, and points of pride.

In the first instances of devaluation, you might interpret bold meanness as constructive criticism, as you aren't prepared for anything other than positive reinforcement. You simply feel that your partner is being awkwardly open, when in fact the narcissist is being intentionally rude. This evokes cognitive dissonance in you, a feeling of mental discomfort that arises when you hold two or more contradictory beliefs simultaneously. In this case, you *know* that the narc is being horrible but you refuse to believe it. Your misconceptions and cognitive dissonance will increase as the narcissist devalues you more and more.

In the beginning, the narcissist exploits your strengths and takes inventory of the qualities you possess, as this will later aid them in manipulating you. They zoom in on your vulnerabilities while preying on your resilience and empathy. In this phase, you feel very alone and confused, but you can't pinpoint the problem. The narcissist starts to withdraw their attention: They stop calling as often or no longer pick up when you call; they don't shower you with compliments but instead flirt or interact playfully with others while barely—or not at all—interacting with you. The love and passion seem to have spilled over to anyone else but you, leaving you feeling lonely, sad, confused, and no longer cherished. Simultaneously, more hurtful behaviors of the narc come creeping in: criticism, hate, disappearing acts, attacks, and any other stressful behavior, such as indiscretion or even infidelity.

Anyone who has ever dealt with narcissistic abuse will remember that very first moment they knew, that exact point in time: "This is the beginning of the end." In my practice, I call it "the first problem in paradise"—the first fracture in the fantastic facade. It's the first moment of devaluation that is *so* blatant, you can't ignore it. "Why would they do this?" always starts with a nasty punch-to-the-gut feeling. It's when the first red flag appears in front of your eyes and you can't deny it. That first moment is the start of the shift from flying on cloud nine to falling into the painful reality of emotional abuse. The extreme change in your partner's behavior will slowly start killing your spirit day by day, month by month, and for some, year by year. It will also start making you physically sick.

From the narcissist's point of view, you stop acting the way they want you to. You might question them for once, actually yell back, call them out on their indiscretion, or be obviously irritated. They don't like this; it annoys them. *Once they feel you act "faulty," they are reminded that they themselves aren't perfect after all, and it is so hurtful that it leaves them angry at you for destroying their idealistic fantasy.* All of a sudden, the everyday emotions feel normal instead of ecstatic—not enough to match their high expectations. Suddenly they start pulling back on their love and affection even more and pushing forward with humiliation, blatant meanness, and hurtful comparisons.

Gaby's Story

"The devaluing phase was what made me disconnect from my true self and lose my essence for a very long time. Something my narcissistic ex-boyfriend once 'loved and admired' about me was that I always saw the good in people. I had no malice in me and that made me somewhat naive, very friendly with everyone. But later he shamed me for it, blaming me for attracting attention from other men because I was 'too good' of a person. He made me believe I was the problem and that I needed to change the very qualities I loved most about myself. Because of my naivety, I let him manipulate me into thinking I had to change, and in doing so, I lost myself and my spark completely."

This treatment begins to cultivate feelings of worthlessness within you. On their way down, narcissists withdraw completely, dragging everyone and everything along in their collapse. They enjoy hurting you, provoking you, setting out to make you the "crazy one" by purposely misplacing things, lying for no reason, or humiliating you in front of relatives and friends. All these attempts to weaken you are usually followed by sweet talk, apologetic behavior, and cuteness to lure you back in, making you believe it isn't so bad after all and you are overreacting. At this point in the relationship, stonewalling and gaslighting play an important role in the dynamics.

Ellie Lisitsa, a clinical psychologist and former staff writer at the Gottman Institute, explains that stonewalling happens when the listener disengages from the conversation, shuts down, and consistently refuses to reengage. It's a challenging behavior to address. Lisitsa, relying on the work of world-renowned psychotherapist and marriage expert John Gottman, clarifies that this destructive pattern of communication is almost a certain guarantee for marital failure. These stonewalling phases consist of stone-cold silences that are undeniably obliterating: You feel invisible to the one you love; you long to bring back a feeling of happiness that seems to have slipped through your fingers.

In addition to stonewalling, narcissists use gaslighting as a tactic. Gaslighting, as explained earlier, is a psychological manipulation technique aimed at planting doubt in a targeted individual, causing them to question their own memory, perception, and sanity. Through persistent denial, misdirection, contradiction, and lying, a narcissist uses gaslighting to destabilize and undermine your beliefs.

Gabriella's Story

"He began pointing out my faults, telling me I was doing things wrong, but he framed his judgments as if they were meant to help us grow together. It sounded reasonable, but it was confusing because many of his criticisms didn't fit me or my situation. He blamed my inconsistent routine for our imbalanced relationship and for any negative emotions I experienced. According to him, my work schedule was the reason I misunderstood him—not his negativity or hurtful behavior. When I asked him to explain what was wrong, he'd respond with vague accusations, such as 'You were so disrespectful' or 'You don't know how to love.' I would ask, 'Okay, please tell me why I wasn't respectful. What made you feel this way?' His response was always dismissive: 'Come on, you were there, you should know.' I'd ask again, 'Please express

yourself more clearly. Help me understand.' But he'd just say, 'When you realize what you did and how you treat me, that will be the beginning of your improvement.' The lack of effective communication and his constant blame left me feeling frustrated and lost."

At this point in the relationship with a narcissist, you come to realize that the person from the honeymoon phase doesn't actually exist. This is an excruciating experience for anyone to have because you have fully invested your mind, heart, and hope in the relationship. Devalued to pieces, you endure relentless verbal and emotional abuse from your narcissistic partner, which leaves you deeply wounded. This abuse infiltrates your mind with disempowering beliefs and messages that undermine your sense of self-worth piece by piece.

This hot-and-cold phase with invalidating emotions causes you to struggle hard. The ice-cold stonewalling is usually accompanied by belittling or ridiculing—when alone or in front of others—and the power struggle doesn't seem to have an end. Usually you are fully aware of what is going on and reluctant to let anyone in on the full truth, as you are embarrassed about being treated this way, which isolates you even more. Most people will not share their experiences for a while because sharing makes it reality. Also, most partners try to protect their narcissist for as long as they can.

Willow's Story
"We reached the point where he found someone new (though I still didn't fully understand what was happening), and the devaluing of me accelerated. Suddenly I wasn't independent enough, I didn't take good enough care of myself, I didn't make enough time for him, I was old and boring. He claimed I spent too much time on myself (I really didn't), questioned why I didn't work more, why the house wasn't cleaner, why I wasn't 'classy' enough (still not sure what he meant by that), why I wasn't less inhibited, why I wanted to talk about sex, why I didn't want to talk about sex, why the kids weren't better behaved, why I wasn't more excited to see him when he got home, and why I didn't just let him come home whenever he wanted. It's important to note that I tried to respond to each of these criticisms with full sincerity—I tried to 'fix' each one. I spent so much energy trying to walk an increasingly narrow tightrope, desperately attempting to be what he wanted. Yet, no matter what I did, it was always wrong. It was either too much or not enough. 'Why are you trying so hard?' 'Why aren't you trying harder?' 'Why don't you just

know what I want?' During all of this, I was trying so hard to fix things because I could sense something was really wrong. I tried couples therapy, I tried initiating sex, I tried backing off about sex. I initiated dates, then I gave him space. I tried to show him I missed him, then I tried not showing it. I asked him what we could do to reconnect. I even asked if he was having an affair (which he was), but he denied it and called me crazy and paranoid. He sat next to me in couples therapy, explaining to our therapist that the issue was with me and that we needed to address my trust issues or else it would ruin our marriage."

Realizing all this is happening to you hits you hard, emotionally and physically. The heartache stemming from the narcissist suddenly withdrawing their love and attention is excruciating; you can't describe it to a person who has never experienced it. It's annihilating. There is this sense of desperation to make it work, and you will try anything and everything in your power to get them to empathize with you, just as Gabriella and Willow did. And you will fail.

Non-abused people can't relate, and this can be quite dangerous when you share your story. If you tell the wrong people (including professionals not trained on emotional abuse), they might reinforce your self-doubt because they can't grasp the depth of emotional abuse, and examples by themselves might seem "pathetic" or "not drastic enough" to cause the hurt you're experiencing. Narcissistic abuse is a lot about context—the how rather than the what.

To ensure control and not fully lose your trust at this point, every now and then the narcissist will add a glimpse of kindness into the mix. This is done so you don't give up the fight completely; they want you to cling to every crumb of hope that you're being handed. This is when intermittent reinforcement begins. You start to be thankful for the breadcrumbs of affection, although that should be a given in any decent relationship. Due to the circumstances, the most basic sign of respect, a positive or neutral gesture, is overappreciated by you, and hope rises again for things to change for the better. *Once you find yourself in a cycle of intermittent reinforcement, your partner holds the position of complete power.* This type of reinforcement is almost always present in a narcissistic relationship. They manage to give you just enough hope for you to stay. They manage to give you just enough kindness and praise for you to think they truly love and care about you. Yet all the while they hold the power and you are left feeling exhausted and defeated.

Right now you're probably thinking that you can't deal with this anymore but you definitely can't leave them either. You're stuck in the worst kind of limbo, fully aware of the slim chances of this working out while still clinging to all your hope. There is this relentless ache permeating every. single. aspect. of your life.

During the difficult phases or bad-mood days of your abuser, you might even experience physical symptoms. You might wake up nauseous with no energy, no matter how long you've slept. Your face might be swollen and pale, no matter how much sun you get. You have a knot in your stomach that doesn't fully allow you to be hungry. You're always on edge. You feel like a shadow of yourself. You might have trouble falling asleep even though you're exhausted. You might experience heightened anxiety that doesn't calm down because you never know what is going to happen next and which version of Dr. Jekyll and Mr. Hyde you are going to meet at home each day. You might have night terrors or nightmares or wake up frequently at night to go to the bathroom. There is a lump in your throat that never seems to leave. You're worried anything could trigger your partner again. It feels cold next to them when it's the middle of a hot summer, and it feels like you're starving even though there's a full bowl of food. It's like reaching for a hand that always pulls away at the last second. It's a constant feeling of not being good enough, of failing at something you can't fully understand in the first place. And the worst part is you can only share this pain with yourself, as your abuser doesn't care about you or your issues.

Whether you feel "strong" enough to endure this phase or too weak to leave, you now enter the next stage—the discarding phase.

3. discard

This is the point where you feel rejected and discarded, or defeated from outright betrayal. The discarding phase is often referred to as the final stage. This is strictly theoretical, as relationships with narcissists rarely have a clean ending but rather an ever-continuing relapse phase where you continue to go back to the perpetrator many times over and over again, often with days or weeks in between, but many times for months and even years.

After you've been discarded, many of your questions are left unanswered and typically you have received no closure. At this point you're most likely so confused that it's overwhelming. You might find yourself replaying conversations, asking yourself, "Was I asking too much?" "Why am I so needy?" "Was I overreacting?" "Did I say it too harshly?" You'll try to pinpoint what caused the switch in their demeanor, to find out where it all went wrong.

The frantic search for answers has you not recognizing yourself. At this point you are questioning your intuition and have most likely turned to your friends for help. You've asked them to analyze every one of the narc's actions. You might have reconstructed fights and obsessed over the meaning of their messages. You find yourself playing detective, compulsively acting out. You may have even gone to the length of secretly recording your conversations with them to replay later as a form of reassurance that you are not insane. You may have done things you are ashamed of, such as stalking their social media or following their car to find the truth behind their lies and deceit.

What you are actually doing is trying to make sense of what happened, where it all went wrong, where *you* went wrong. Yet you're not able to settle for any satisfying answer. All you find is a nasty, gnawing, and disturbing sense of self-doubt. Any self-confidence you once had is drowned out as their voice of doubt and judgment inside your head grows louder. Their voice can make you believe you are not worthy and the things they have been telling you are actually true. You might hear their voice in your head saying things like, "Look at you, you look like an absolute wreck!" or "You are so lucky to have me" or "You won't find anyone who will love you like I did." And you truly believe them.

Tom's Story

"There were plenty of things she said to me. She used phrases like, 'No one will love you like I do; you are no one' or 'Don't forget, I am rich, and you need me.' She would shout things like, 'I am the attractive and charismatic one, not you!' She told me that's why I would end up dying alone. After months of horrible abuse and being left bereft of all joy, I started believing her from the bottom of my heart."

This is naturally the most painful and humiliating stage, as all your loyalty toward your narc didn't pay off. You feel physically exhausted, cognitively confused, and emotionally devastated. Usually this phase only takes place when the narcissist has found another "target" to cling to and has decided to let you go—often slowly, without the intent to stop torturing you yet. They will rub other possible partners in your face and, at the same time, deny that they are cheating. They'll tell you you're crazy, jealous, or both. If they have met someone that they can start sucking dry instead of you, they love to show it off. They will flaunt their new supply in your face, leaving you feeling like you never meant anything to them. You will be thinking things like, "Did I ever mean anything to them if they can just move on and be happy with someone else so quickly?" and "How can they just leave me that easily after all the promises they made to me?"

Suzy's Story

"He started coming home from work late, often very drunk and smelling of perfume. Our date nights became rare as he spent more time going out with friends and taking multiple trips with the guys. Often he wouldn't come home until after 3 a.m. on weekends, and he behaved strangely when he did. I felt more alone when I was with him than when I was actually by myself."

You still can't grasp the reality of it all: "It was so easy and fun, light and loving, just two weeks ago, just yesterday. Where has all that gone? Who is this person? Why are they switching back and forth? Where is the person I fell in love with?" When you give them two options, they say no to both but won't let you have a third option. *It's lose-lose with a narcissist. You will never win.* You feel isolated and alone, trapped in a nightmare where the person who once made you feel so loved now seems set on destroying you. And they are.

Synthia's Story

"Without warning, after all this time of saying I was the love of his life, talking about building a home together, marriage, and having babies, he ended the relationship through a WhatsApp message, leaving me devastated and feeling completely discarded. After everything we had planned together, he simply walked away and never looked back as if none of it had ever happened. Despite all the love and trust I had placed in him, when his mask fell off, there was nothing left."

4. destroy

The narc is now switching from the person who made you feel complete to the person who tears away your life energy source with every single thing they do.

It's literally emotional whiplash. You might still be in shock from digesting what is actually happening to you. The now so obviously sharp contrast from "their perfect self" to "their psychopathic self" devastates you like a car accident that just happened. It seems surreal.

The destroy phase is when the narcissist feels you're no longer a good supply to them and they want to practice a sort of "revenge" on you. They can't stand seeing that you're okay—or God forbid, happy—without them, so they spend a substantial amount of energy on destroying you. They destroy you with seemingly no effort, guilt, or shame in order to feel better about themselves. The destroy phase also acts as prevention. It's their way of stopping you from exposing how horrible they are, because you will be so preoccupied with picking up your own pieces. This makes it easier for them to call you crazy, as you will seemingly be "crazy" during this phase. You may act like a psychological wreck and not look put together, perhaps not taking care of simple things such as hygiene, as you obsess over the narc's behavior. People in your life might be asking why you are so preoccupied with and despondent over the narc if they are as bad as you say. It won't make sense from the outside. You will seem delusional. That's exactly what the narc wants. They want to win this sick foul play.

As a result, you are often left with massive trauma (called complex post-traumatic stress disorder, C-PTSD, which we will discuss later), not understanding the heartless indifference with which you are exchanged for another supply. You feel disposed of (and you are), like a piece of trash. You used to think the narcissist loved you, but now all you do is doubt. At this point, the narc has you right where they need you to be— believing what they've said to you all along: "The only problem here is you." The destroy phase leaves you feeling empty, depressed, and, worst of all, hopeless.

Lola's Story
"Whenever I cried because of him, he would become annoyed and aggressive, telling me not to 'cry like a little bitch.' It was heartbreaking to watch his eyes turn ice-cold during arguments and to feel the incredible indifference he radiated. I fought, bawled my eyes out, and explained myself—so full of love, pouring all my energy into him, just to restore things to how they used to be. He did absolutely nothing in return and blamed me for everything that went wrong. He lived like a bachelor, justifying it by saying I lacked a sense of togetherness. He was secretly seeing his ex-wife, but my jealousy was supposedly what ruined everything. He lied to me

repeatedly, and when I once answered his cell phone, he said the relationship was over because he wouldn't be controlled. He never took responsibility for his actions and always left me feeling guilty."

In addition to the internal war you're experiencing, the outside world may now be a war zone as well, as the narcissist will not stop trying to destroy you. Other people will have a hard time believing you and often won't understand what you're going through. If you have dared to tell people around you about your relationship problems, you probably won't continue for very long. If you decide to keep people updated with a live ticker, you'll spend hours a day on the phone ruminating about what new toxic situation has occurred; and people will say, "Honey, this is ridiculous" or "Gosh, well, if it's so bad, you should just leave them. Why are you still here?!" No matter what they say, they will not be able to help you feel differently about your abuser. Not only will you hear unhelpful comments like this, but this phase might include being extremely disappointed with the people around you whom you thought you could confide in but actually can't. You thought these people had your back, and now they might even seem to be siding with the narc.

Ethan's Story

"Since I left her, she made sure I paid for it. I found out she was flirting with one of my closest friends, and within two weeks she was out with other guys, posting pictures like I never existed, telling people I wasn't good enough for her, that I didn't make enough money to keep her happy. This was the same woman who, just a month earlier, told me I was the love of her life, that she couldn't imagine being with anyone else. Now she's acting like I never mattered, and all those words feel like nothing but empty promises."

You may start to feel like an absolute fool because the circus never ends. You find yourself swaying back and forth between moments of manic happiness, clinging to a string of hope they throw at you, and then feeling totally depressed, confused, numb, and empty like a hollow shell. The destroy phase may come with a disturbing turn of events, revealing shocking truths about the depth of the narcissist's betrayals or an especially intense outburst of rage. It can also hit you out of nowhere. Regardless of how the destroy phase unfolds, it is ruthless and deliberately intended to cause you harm.

The harm of the destroy phase is felt not only psychologically but also physically. You might experience subtle things such as constant exhaustion, dizziness, or agitation on a higher level. You might experience reoccurring headaches, throat infections, gastrointestinal issues, or skin rashes. Worse and more intense signs could be your hair falling out, drastic changes in libido, irregular menstrual cycles for women, or impotence for men.

B's Story

"Eventually, after he pushed me down for the second time, I called the police. That was the moment he was done with me. It was like flipping a switch—every shred of love and kindness he had once shown me was gone in an instant. He said he could never be with someone who would call the police on him, no matter what he'd done. He insisted it was all my fault, claiming I'd made it all up and 'ruined everything.' After that, the discard was complete, and he began trying to destroy me. He told anyone who would listen that the failure of our marriage was entirely my fault—I was crazy, spent too much money, and was controlling. He said no wonder he'd cheated, that he'd never loved me and had only stayed for the kids. Whenever I shared my experiences in the marriage, he would attack, portraying himself as the victim of slander, while I was simply sharing the facts of what had happened. He took money from our shared account, then removed himself from it, leaving me with the bills. He made financial agreements with me, both verbally and in writing, then later denied they existed, putting me in one difficult financial situation after another. Now he's fighting me in court for every possible dime, lying that we had an open marriage and claiming I was a terrible wife, blaming me for the breakdown of our marriage."

You might not have been knowledgeable about the abuse cycle and tactics of a narcissist at this point and, due to this, blame yourself for not being good enough. You feel it is your fault—your fault that you are being abused, and your fault that you keep staying—and your self-worth is at an all-time low. During this phase, unless you allow the narcissist to lure you back into another cycle, you are able to start healing. Healing is simply surviving at this point. If you let them lure you back in, the abuse cycle restarts itself and you are again caught up in a traumatic relationship spiral. You won't be feeling less sad, less scared, less addicted, less frustrated, less angry with yourself, or less fragile unless *you* put in the work to ensure you never go back or let them lure you back in the next phase.

5. hoover

Hoovering is the phase after the end of the relationship. Because narcissists always need to stay in control and leave nothing up to you or fate, they need to control how it ends as well. If you had the audacity to leave them, they will do everything in their power to get you back—just to break up with you after. They want to finish the relationship on their terms, not yours.

K's Story

"After I finally built up the strength to leave him, he tried to pull me back in. He suggested couples therapy, and I agreed, hoping against hope that we could find a way to make it work for the sake of our daughter. But even in therapy, he lied straight to the therapist's face, twisting the truth to make himself look like the victim and me the unreasonable one. It became clear that nothing would change."

Hoovering is just another awful manipulation tactic. It is when the narcissist revolves around you like a Hoover (vacuum) to lure you back into the cyclone of destructive dependence. The narcissist attempts to win you back by being charming and sweet. They send presents, apologize; they act courteous, angry, or upset, threatening suicide or self-harm; they may sit in front of your house every night, crying. They will do anything they can whisk out of their little magic hat. They try these tactics hoping that you end up falling for one of them, only to be caught up in their web of terror once more.

Ava's Story

"He messaged me five months after we ended things, telling me he loved me so much, apologizing and saying he regretted everything. I'd been waiting to hear those words for months, so I responded right away, hoping maybe this time he meant it. He brought up old memories, asked if I missed him, and suggested we meet up. I knew I shouldn't, but I agreed, hoping maybe things had finally changed and he understood what he had lost. I waited at the café, but he never showed up. When I then called him, he answered his phone very annoyed, saying that I just woke him up from his nap for nothing and wasted his time, and then he hung up. I felt like a complete idiot. I realized I'd fallen for it all over again—absolutely nothing was different. I felt like a fool. I had reopened wounds that were finally starting to heal, and I was left hurting all over again. It felt like it hurt more than the first time around."

Of course, whenever any relationship ends, there might be some back-and-forth or an aftermath to the story. That is to be expected. People will realize that they made mistakes, apologize, try to get their partner back, and make promises to change. In a healthy relationship, it's when partners realize that things went wrong and they want to truly work on the relationship and change. The key difference to the narcissist's hoovering is that they have no intention of changing. I call it NATO (no action, talk only) and nothing, absolutely nothing, will ever change.

Ryan's Story

"Every time she came back, I'd convince myself it was different. She'd say she missed me, and I'd fall for it, like an idiot, thinking maybe this time she really meant it. But deep down, I knew something wasn't right. It wasn't love—something was off, something that always left me feeling worse after she pulled me back in. I'd regret it the moment I gave in, hating myself for always going back, but I couldn't help it. She had this hold over me, and I kept hoping she'd be the person I wanted her to be, even though every time she left me more broken than before."

CHECK-IN

Take a moment to reflect on how you have experienced the five phases of abuse in your own life. What did your partner do to make you feel small or powerless? What was the hardest part for you when you tried to leave? Was there something that made it feel impossible at the time? Think about how the hoovering phase played out in your situation. What patterns or tactics did the narcissist use to try to pull you back in? Now consider what has worked/works best for you to resist their attempts. You've already come so far by recognizing the cycle. What's the next step for you?

where to go from here

Any survivor of narcissistic abuse has felt this cycle play out several times in their relationship. The phases of hope are surpassed by the disappointment of them again not trying to change, and it is extremely painful to live through. It feels as though someone is deliberately torturing you, which they are. At this point, survivors often become so full of rage that they turn against themselves. This can fester in random acts of self-sabotage, such as negative self-talk, treating your body poorly, and doing things that don't serve you. You may find yourself overreacting to any little provocation from the narc, as you are quite destabilized in this fragile period. Your possible overreactions during this time will be held against you. You will continually be blamed for the relationship not working. When they are finally ready to bounce again, they leave you abruptly, out of the blue, with no adequate reason, no explanation, and no closure. *Now* they feel ready, and suddenly they decide to discard you like a piece of trash, for the last time.

The abuse cycle has lasting impacts. Even if you are not carrying visible bruises on the outside, you will feel invisible wounds, physically and mentally. Your body might not be functioning like it used to, your hair might be falling out, you might not recognize the person staring back at you in the mirror. You are most likely suffering from post-traumatic stress, and you might feel emotionally unstable. All this is very common, and you are not alone. Step by step and day by day there are things you can do to heal.

From personal and professional experience of leaving a narcissist, I have many useful lessons to share with you. Going forward in this book, I will share everything I know about the aftermath of leaving them and the path of healing. I hope the concepts and therapeutic insights you learned in this chapter will help you accept what has happened. The cycle of the narc's abuse can make your head spin, making you feel crazy. But narcissists have remarkably similar traits and use specific tactics to manipulate and control their relationships, which we'll examine in the next chapter. Prepare to have your blurry vision come into clearer focus.

chapter 3

you are not crazy (even if you feel crazy right now)

"A narcissist is someone who sticks their head
up their own ass, then blames you for the smell."

—Steve Maraboli

In the first chapters, I explained what exactly a narcissistic partner is and what their abuse cycle entails. We have established that you must be feeling horrible, empty, and desperate right now. What we have not yet discussed is the question that every survivor asks themselves after going through all these mind manipulations: "Am I the crazy one? Am I the narcissist?!" I can tell you that not a single survivor of narc abuse is immune to this question, as you have been gaslit into thinking that you are the defective one, not them. It is a perfectly healthy sign of reflection and self-awareness that proves you are not the crazy one or a narcissist, because a narcissist would never ask themselves these questions.

The renowned German writer Johann Wolfgang von Goethe wrote that often we have two souls living in our heart, conveying the internal conflict of two contradictory beliefs or loyalties. When abuse survivors ask me, as a therapist, if they are the narcissist, I notice exactly that: two hearts beating in my chest. One heart sighs with relief, recognizing that the person in front of me is capable of reflecting and surely not a narcissist. The other heart falls deep into the core of my stomach, as it confirms the abuse they've endured and its damaging effects.

What do I mean by "damaging effects"? There are classic tactics every narcissist uses throughout their relationships and quite frankly the entire abuse cycle. The goal of all these tactics is always the same: *to maintain power over you and make you doubt yourself*. The more self-doubt they plant in you, the more power and control they gain. With these tactics they constantly insinuate that you are weak, stupid, slow, ugly, small. They tell you that you are a bad person, an awful parent, a crappy sibling, a horrible friend—the list goes on. The damaging effects begin to take hold when you're exposed to these horrible insults repeatedly over long periods of time. After a while, whether you want to or not, you start to believe them and you start complying.

twenty-four toxic traits

The good news is that narcissists are copy/paste. You *can* basically predict their behavior if you know all their tricks and deceit mechanisms. For you to be one step ahead, I will describe twenty-four toxic traits of a narcissist so you can recognize them right away.

1. they idealize and love-bomb you

The first toxic trait to look out for is the first phase in the abuse cycle, which we covered in chapter 2: idealization and love-bombing. As previously described, the narcissist will shower you with praise and give you endless compliments, making you feel like a million bucks at all times. They will use social media to shower you with their attention, complimenting all your photos, sending you random cute messages and funny memes, posting positive things about you, and writing captions like "Love of my life" underneath your pictures. This will have you melting from their sweetness. The sugar they sprinkle you with is all a tactic: It is designed to manipulate you to become addicted to their constant attention.

To help you spot this toxic trait, pay attention to their kindness and attentiveness, as their focus on you is 24/7. They communicate with you constantly. You receive good-morning calls and goodnight texts and fifty texts in between. They call you nonstop to check in on you, see how you're doing, how you're feeling, and if there is anything they can do to brighten your day. They send you updates on their every move and every new felt emotion, as simple as "I was so happy that my colleague put gummi bears in the kitchen!" They will drive you places and pick you up, come over daily, cook for you, spoil you, and make love to you any chance they get. They will compliment you, be proud of you, love your decisions and your character and flaunt this to you and everyone else, raise you on a pedestal, and adore the ground you walk on. This all seems extremely sweet and cute, and you will get used to their constant obsession very quickly. But beware: They are *not* doing this because they love you so endlessly. They are doing it to create the illusion that you are seen and loved and completed by them. Their attention feels so special that you will become fully dependent on it. That is exactly what they want. They want you to need them.

2. they stonewall you

The second toxic trait is stonewalling, when they put an invisible but dramatic "wall of stone" between you and them, which translates into you being completely ignored. When you do something for the first time that does not align with the narc's requirements, expect to be punished for it. Either they will direct their aggression at you by yelling at or devaluing you, or they will stonewall you. This will feel like it is happening out of nowhere, but it isn't. It's the first irritation you give them—the first time you're not the perfect puppet in their show. It's the first time you question them, criticize them, or ask something of them—and they don't like it. Their reaction will be blown way out of proportion, and you will be baffled. You might even think that they're kidding—but they're serious. This is their way of grooming you to understand everything needs to go their way. You can expect a gentle form of stonewalling, one that only lasts for some minutes or perhaps hours within the first month of dating them. After that, it gets worse every time and becomes longer and colder, sometimes lasting weeks on end where they completely ignore you.

Stonewalling is the exact opposite of idealization and love-bombing. If a partner stonewalls you, you are receiving the opposite of attention: You are being ignored. They will use this whenever you engage in any behavior that they do not appreciate. Perhaps you ask questions about their offensive behavior. If they feel offended by those questions (very likely) or even deem them as invasive, they will punish you by ignoring you. If you did something they don't appreciate, instead of letting you know, they will turn to stonewalling without an explanation. The "thing" you did can be as small as buying them the wrong shower gel or not closing your eyes when you kissed them goodbye. They also use this when you don't do something they want.

This is not a typical spur-of-the-moment reaction where someone needs space because they are upset. The narc will ignore you for hours, days, or even weeks at a time and will not let you know why. This is literally a torture method they use to make you feel extremely isolated and guilty. They will stonewall you through their body language as well. They might turn their shoulders away, avoid eye contact, cross their arms and legs, and position their body away from you during dinner. This passive-aggressive behavior only shows their frustration but doesn't try to resolve tension, which is what a healthy partner would strive for. Healthy partners would communicate their reasons for being upset in a healthy manner. The reason the narc does not do this is because they are mostly not *actually* upset by the course of events but rather looking for ways to punish you. It is a game for them to drive you crazy and thus weaken you for them to gain more power and control, and they actually enjoy it.

A narcissist uses this tactic to make you feel insecure and extremely confused. You will be left not knowing or understanding what you did or what just happened to cause such an intense reaction. Stonewalling, in short, is their blatant refusal to engage or cooperate.

3. they triangulate you

The third toxic trait is triangulation. Triangulation occurs when the narcissist creates a "triangle" involving you, them, and another person (or more). They involve people you love and are close to; they may falsely claim that these individuals have said something bad about you. In narc lingo we call the people they use in triangulation "flying monkeys." This tactic is particularly malicious because their intention is to harm you emotionally and make you doubt your connection with your loved ones. The goal is to make you question the loyalty of all the people around you that you care about. This may be your parent, sibling, best friend, work colleague, or sports coach. The narcissist might say things like, "You know your best friend said you looked really bad in that outfit?" You think, "Why would my best friend say that? That does not sound like them." But you are quite hurt on the inside, and disappointment starts to build. The reality is the best friend never said that.

Another example might be your narcissistic partner telling you that your mother said you acted entitled during last weekend's brunch with everyone. They are planting a seed in your mind, making you wonder, "Why is everybody against me?" That is exactly what they strive for. The less you are in touch with your family and friends, the easier you are to control and even coerce.

This is a deliberate tactic to isolate you. Once you begin to doubt and become skeptical of the people you consider close to you, you may start to isolate yourself without the pressure of your abuser. You withdraw on your own from everyone you trust, and you think to yourself, "The only person I can trust is them [your abuser]." This is exactly where the narcissist wants you—alone with them—no one there to tell you that whatever is happening is toxic; no one to remind you of all the stunts your narcissist has pulled; no one to mirror how tired you seem to look lately; and no one to tell you how what happened the other day is *not* okay.

It is very important to recognize triangulation as abuse. If you do not recognize that you are being triangulated with the people you love, you risk being isolated with your narcissistic partner. If you are isolated with them, they have the perfect opportunity to exert more power over you. If you are unsure if triangulation is occurring, make it a point to ask your loved ones about the narc's claims and cross-check with them for validation. If all of them say that it never happened, perhaps it's enough proof that the narc is lying.

CHECK-IN

Think back to the times the narc told you that someone you cared about allegedly said bad things about you. Then ask yourself whether you simply believed the narc was telling the truth or whether you verified the allegations by confronting that person. If you didn't verify it, get in touch with the person and ask them about it.

break up with narcissism

Of course, ordinary people lie too, and your best friend could have been caught gossiping about you, or your sports trainer might have said something not nice behind your back and then not told you the truth when you confronted them. So in the end, you might doubt some people and think the narc was actually telling the truth. The people around you don't always have your back; they are not always honest and morally correct. People do lie and gossip—that's natural. But if, since you've paired up with Mr. or Ms. Narc, everyone suddenly seems dodgy and is badmouthing you all the time, then you should become suspicious and question the narc, not your friends and loved ones.

Another classic triangulation tactic is when they tell you about all the "crazy" people in their lives. For instance, this could be an ex-partner, an ex-boss, a former client, or anyone they had to deal with. Your natural reaction might be to think, "Oh, that person is crazy, so you're no longer spending time with them." But let me tell you, you thought wrong. In reality, they continue to spend time with these "crazy" people, causing you to doubt your memory. You wonder, "Why are you hanging out with this person? I don't understand." The narcissist does this because it gives them the power to make you feel crazy and an opportunity to devalue you for judging them for hanging out with these "crazy" people. For instance, they might say things like, "What's wrong with you? Are you jealous? Why are you being like that? Don't be so clingy and needy." This will leave you feeling as if you are in an endless circle of insanity. It won't make sense, and it will leave you questioning your sense of reality even more.

Also, triangulation will make you feel more and more like an outsider in the narc's life. They continue to spend time with people they claim to dislike while reducing the time they spend with you. You will be left in the dark, on the outside, not a part of that group. It will feel like your partner values this group of "crazy" people more than they value you. Ultimately all this triangulation will naturally lead you to question your own memory and judgment.

Here's a dialogue inspired by Nina's story:

> **NINA:** *You've been spending a lot of time with your colleague Sarah lately. I feel like you're spending more time after work with her than with me, and I'm confused. Didn't you tell me she was obsessed with you and it creeped you out?*

NARCISSIST: *Sarah? Obsessed? No, that was just in the beginning. She's always been supportive and so kind. She actually cares how I am doing and always stays in touch. Maybe if you were more like her, I wouldn't spend so much time with her after work.*

NINA: *That's hurtful. I'm trying my best to be there for you, but you're never around. I make dinners and you don't show up. It really makes me feel lonely.*

NARCISSIST: *Oh, come on, don't be so dramatic. Sarah just cooks better than you do. It's not her fault if you're insecure about your cooking. You're just overreacting. Sarah never makes me feel guilty like this.*

4. they gaslight you

Gaslighting is a technique narcissists use to drive you insane by making you question reality. The narcissist will constantly make you feel crazy by planting doubt in your mind about things that happened and then pretending that they didn't. They will also deny things they said that you know for sure were said. For example, your partner might text you that they're going to the gym, but in reality they're spending time with a friend. On its own, hanging out with a friend is not a big deal. But when you find out that they are hanging out with their friend rather than actually at the gym, it is distressing. You're left questioning reality: "Why would they tell me they are at the gym when they are spending time with their friends?"

It is understandable that this statement wouldn't make sense to you. You are right to feel confused. It leaves so much space for your imagination to run wild. It does not make any sense, and it shouldn't, as it is not normal. The point of gaslighting is to drive you crazy, to make you think you're losing your mind. The kicker is that if you confront the narc with proof of their lie, they'll turn it around and say, "It's not a big deal! Why are you making such a big deal out of me hanging out with my friend?" They will dramatize your reaction, even though they are blatantly lying to you. When a narcissistic partner continues to gaslight you, it can lead to heightened vigilance and hypersensitivity, even though this is not reflective of your true nature. I call that "trying to make sense of crazy will drive you insane." You will find yourself with thoughts that are unlike you, doing things you normally would never do out of desperation (playing detective, screaming, even getting physical).

They will continue to gaslight you until you believe their behavior is your fault—even if it sounds ridiculous! While in this type of relationship, you will start to genuinely believe everything they say despite remembering things correctly and often even having proof of the matter. This makes you doubt your own sense of reality and self-efficacy. The gaslighting further deepens your existing sense of isolation, making you feel unloved and unworthy.

Here's a dialogue inspired by Melissa's story, illustrating gaslighting:

MELISSA: *I found a pair of women's underwear in our bedroom. How could you bring her here while the kids and I were away?*

NARCISSIST: *What are you talking about? I didn't bring anyone here. You're imagining things.*

MELISSA: *But I found them on our floor. You admitted she was here before!*

NARCISSIST: *Yes, she stopped by for a minute, but those aren't hers. They're probably yours and you don't remember. You're being paranoid—thinking up wild stories. Do you even hear yourself?*

MELISSA: *I'm not imagining it! They're not mine. I would know. How can you now blatantly deny what you already admitted? Stop lying and just tell me you're sleeping with her in our bed again.*

NARCISSIST: *Lied? You're the one twisting this. You're always looking for reasons to start a fight. It's exhausting, honestly. You're so insecure it's almost sad. Maybe you should talk to someone about these trust issues.*

Here are some common gaslighting phrases that my clients report:

"Look what you made me do."

"You're being too sensitive."

"You're the only person that has a problem with this."

"Everyone else agrees with me."

"I was just joking. You are taking it too seriously."

"You're remembering it wrong."

"No one else will love you like I do."

"No, I didn't send that text/take that picture/speak to that person."

5. they are charming with everyone else but you

A narcissist will conceal their true colors in the company of others, only revealing their authentic nature when they are alone with you. You will be the only witness to their manipulation tactics and treatment of you. There is a reason that you are the only person who sees their true colors. Only when they start to feel comfortable and know that they have you in their pocket will they reveal who they really are. This control makes them feel secure enough to use you as the punching bag on which to take out all their frustrations and insecurities. They don't want others to notice their fakeness, their issues, their flaws. They'd never want their mask to fall off and reveal their flawed self in front of others. For everyone else they keep up the facade to maintain their perfect image: They have to stay charming and beautiful, sweet and cute, completely charismatic—all those things that they don't have to be with you anymore. The narcissist thrives on external validation, and if other people do not know the narc's true nature, they will give the narc the validation they so endlessly seek.

You have most likely asked yourself, "Why are they being so nice to everyone else but me? Why are they so willing to help others, but when I ask for help, I am accused of being too needy?" The answer is very simple: As long as they keep up their perfect image for others, you will have a much harder time getting anyone to believe that this wonderful person could be abusing you behind closed doors. The narcissist is very aware of every single step they take, and everything they do is perfectly construed to show to whomever they want to show it to. They are manipulative; they know exactly what they are doing. None of it is a coincidence; it's all strategy and agenda.

Reminder: Their behavior is purely their fault.

6. they pathologically lie

Pathological lying is the act of lying constantly without any apparent reason or benefit. Unlike regular lying (that we all sometimes do) where people get something out of it or avoid some sort of unfortunate consequence, pathological lying (only pathological individuals do) seems compulsive and useless. It's astonishing how easily narcissists can lie to you for no reason whatsoever, with a straight face.

Pathological lying often goes hand in hand with gaslighting. It causes you to question your memory and wonder whether you were paying proper attention. Even if you have all the proof in the world, a narcissist will still look you straight in the eyes, lie, and deny everything that just happened.

The word *crazy* keeps coming up because this is exactly how you will feel—like you've gone crazy, like you don't understand them or the world around you. You keep asking yourself, "Why would they do this?" And you can't come up with an answer. You may even go to the lengths of playing detective, following them around to see if what they are doing aligns with what they told you, because you start to doubt your own reality and perception. That doubt is one of the worst parts of being a narcissist's victim—it only fuels your self-hatred even more. You don't know what to believe anymore, even though your gut feeling is screaming at you every single day not to believe them. You can't eat, as your dissonance is eating you alive from the inside and still staying put. Does what they did align with what they told you they did? It usually doesn't. If you then confront them, they will start all over again, blaming you for being absurd, crazy, paranoid, insane, frustrated, or bored. If you fall into this detective role, you will find yourself for weeks on end trying to make sense of it all without closure. *You will never find an answer because trying to make sense of a narcissist's pathological lying is an impossible quest*. This is the tactic they use to further confuse your sense of reality. If you start to notice that your partner (or anyone for this matter!) is constantly lying to you, especially about the smallest irrelevant things, please distance yourself from this person.

A True Story about an Ex-Boyfriend of Mine

Every so often my ex-boyfriend would say to me, "Got called into work—I gotta go."
It was his way of reminding me he was a busy and important doctor, sacrificing personal time for the greater good, always on call. But something about that night didn't sit right with me again—a nasty gut feeling I couldn't ignore anymore. I just constantly felt that he was lying. So, it being the middle of the night, I took a taxi, half-embarrassed by my own suspicions and half-driven by a need to know the truth. Playing detective, I gave the driver his address and held my breath as we approached his house.

And there he was—parked in front of his own home, alone in his car. No scrubs, no pager, no sense of urgency. Just the soft glow of his car light illuminating a book in his lap. I watched, stunned, as he turned a page, completely absorbed. I sat there for a moment in the cab, staring in confusion. It was almost surreal, like a scene you'd accidentally walked into that wasn't meant for you to see. I started crying and laughing simultaneously, thinking to myself, "What the . . . This can't be real." The driver seemed utterly confused. Suddenly I realized that every late-night shift or emergency call was most likely BS. I seriously doubted he was even a doctor at that point. I later found out he was seeing plenty of other women and in fact sleeping with most of his nurses. So, yes, he was a doctor, just not busy saving lives but sleeping around.

CHECK-IN

Make sure you note in your journal every single time that you catch them lying, no matter how small, so you have a list later and won't forget any of it.

---

7. they lack empathy

A narcissist has no empathy. They have no ability to place themselves in your shoes or relate to any feelings you may have. They only have the ability to *fake* empathy when they need to in the beginning phase of your relationship. Whether you're telling them an exciting story, explaining why you're upset or sad, expressing concern about something or someone, or feeling distressed about an animal being mistreated, they are unable to connect with your emotions. They can't and will not be able to empathize with you. No matter how well you articulate something, they are incapable of understanding. It's like describing a color to a blind person. Empathy is a trait they do not have, and they have no interest in learning it because it isn't beneficial to their only goal: to get more power over you and suck you dry. If they were empathetic, that emotion would stand in their way.

You can test their empathy by telling them a very touching story and then observe their reaction closely. The key is to look for a genuine reaction. They might show their fake empathy through soothing words, alligator tears, or a suitable facial expression, but you can see beyond this. They will quickly wrap up their "touched" self and start talking about something else. They might throw out a sob story about themselves to not have to be involved in your story for too long. Either way, be careful here and notice that the narc is just pretending to feel with you. Watch them closely and pay attention to their body language, as that is harder to hide. Narcs are great with words, but not as good with their body language. If your gut is telling you something is off, it is. Within minutes, they will usually fail to continue to ask questions and truly seem interested. They're more likely to brush it off and only tell you a couple of words they believe you want to hear, and then quickly change the topic.

Anita's Story

"The circumstances after the birth of our fourth child were extreme: My husband's mother had to be hospitalized, and our three children were sick with 104°F (40°C) fevers. Since my husband could not risk contaminating his mother, he stayed away, and I took care of three sick children and a newborn, just being out of a C-section three days prior. I was hormonally and emotionally challenged to my breaking point. When my husband came to visit, he found me curled up naked on the bathroom floor, sobbing and in pain. Instead of helping me get dressed and comforting me, he looked down on me, disgusted that I wasn't able to manage better. He screamed, 'You are the worst person I could have married! I wish I had never married you!' He stormed out of the house, leaving me sobbing on the floor, and he didn't come back until the next afternoon, never mentioning the incident again."

8. their mistakes never count

An infuriating toxic trait narcissists carry is refusing to take responsibility for their mistakes. Their mistakes never ever count, while all of yours are a massive deal. No matter what serious mistake they make, they will do anything to turn it around, take no responsibility, and point the finger back at you.

Imagine they forget your birthday and do nothing to celebrate you. When you confront them about it, expressing how much it hurt your feelings, rather than apologizing and owning up to the fact they forgot, they will bring up something from the past to take the attention off them and back onto you. For example:

YOU: *I was really hurt that you forgot my birthday. It felt like you didn't care about celebrating me at all.*

NARCISSIST: *Oh, so now I'm the bad guy? Remember when you showed up late to that dinner we had last year? I didn't make a big deal about it, did I?*

YOU: *But this is different. This was my birthday. I just wanted to feel appreciated.*

NARCISSIST: *I can't believe you're making such a big deal out of this. You're always bringing things up to make me look bad. Maybe if you weren't so sensitive, we wouldn't have these issues.*

YOU: *I'm not being sensitive! It's such a crappy move for a partner to forget my birthday and then not even want to make up for it! Last year you treated me like royalty for my birthday, and now this? Who are you? You haven't even apologized.*

NARCISSIST: *Well, maybe if you were more considerate sometimes, you'd see how hard it is to keep up with everything. But no, it's always about you, isn't it?"*

What's happening here is the narcissist is bringing up any mistake, even a small one that wouldn't be a big deal in a healthy relationship, to justify their own *huge* mistake instead of simply apologizing. They blow these things way out of proportion so that no matter how horrible their mistake is, they can easily dismiss it like it's nothing, because "you have made so many mistakes before."

Remember, a narcissist is very skilled with their words. Even when they are in the wrong, they can make you feel like you're the one blowing things out of proportion and turning a small issue into a big one. When this happens, write down what occurred to remind yourself that you are not at fault, and share the situation with a trusted friend who can also remind you that you're not wrong and that what the narcissist has done is not okay. Trust your instincts.

9. they are beyond selfish

Once you get past their loving facade, you will find a very selfish side. A narcissist will not allow their partner to do the simplest things. They do this because they want to control and maintain the attention around them. Their needs come first. You will eat what they want to eat when they want to eat it, as they dictate food choices and mealtimes. You will go to bed when they want to go to bed, even if you're an early bird and they are a night owl, or vice versa. They will make sure you succumb to their schedule. Obviously you will only go out when they want you to go out, and they will control your company. No more meeting whoever you want without checking in with them. Through all of this, they imply that their needs, routines, and wishes are more important than yours. This has a massive element of disrespect that you may not have noticed yet.

You will find this type of behavior to be very hypocritical. They are allowed to do whatever they want when they want, while you are not allowed to do anything you want unless they give permission. It demonstrates their compulsion to control you and shows their absurd selfishness. The whole world revolves around them.

In case you're unsure how selfish your narc might be, there are easy ways to test it out for yourself. Here are two examples:

1. Plan a weekend activity that you enjoy and that you know your partner isn't too fond of. (For example, if you're an outdoor person and they are a city person, or the other way around.) See whether they are willing to do your activity without complaining every once in a while or try to find a suitable compromise. A narcissist most likely won't be willing and you'll end up doing their preferred activity.

2. When you want your partner to hang out with your friends, but they always choose theirs over yours, it's a red flag for selfishness. Propose a few dates and ideas with your friends and see how the narc reacts. Are they always making up an excuse, seemingly not able to join? If so, they simply don't care enough about your people, and their social circles are more important to them than yours. This is common to some degree, but a healthy partner tries to do both—spend time with their own as well as your friends.

10. they accuse you of feeling emotions they are intentionally provoking

A narcissist will intentionally try to provoke emotions. Again, the narcissist does this to belittle you and therefore gain more control. A classic example is instilling jealousy.

They tell you how superhot and super-fun their ex is while letting you know they plan on going hiking with them. Of course this will make you feel jealous! It would make anyone feel off.

If you express how uncomfortable this makes you, the narcissist uses your "jealousy" against you, calling it inappropriate, dramatic, or unnecessary. If you would dare to do the same, they would freak out, but when it's them doing it, it's okay, and you're the psycho. It is all about playing a game with your mind. They instill jealousy in you, you react appropriately, and then they try to make you feel bad for it by calling your reaction "over the top." This is partly gaslighting, partly triangulating, partly pathological lying (how everyone else is awesome but you are insane), and partly pure evil.

Further examples include telling you something outrageous, intentionally causing you to get angry; instilling sadness and then accusing you of being too sensitive; or instilling feelings of clinginess because they have started to withdraw and then accuse you of being too needy. The list goes on.

Here's a dialogue inspired by Monica's story:

> **MONICA:** *I really don't want to see pictures of your ex. You know it just makes me feel uneasy.*
>
> **NARCISSIST:** *Wow, I didn't think you'd be so uptight about it. She was a big part of my life, you know that.*
>
> **MONICA:** *I get that, but it feels like you're bringing her up on purpose. Why would you want me to feel this way?*
>
> **NARCISSIST:** *(casually scrolling and "accidentally" flashing a photo) Oops—well, there she is. I mean, can you blame me for being with her? She's stunning.*
>
> **MONICA:** *Why do you keep doing this? I asked you not to show me these photos.*
>
> **NARCISSIST:** *Are you seriously getting worked up over a picture? Maybe you need to work on your confidence. It's honestly a turn-off to see you this jealous.*

11. they are always hypocrites

A narcissist is and will always be a nonstop hypocrite. They maintain two separate standards of judging: what is acceptable for them, and what is not acceptable for you; what they are allowed to do, and what you are not allowed to do. For example, they are allowed to go on vacation with their friends, but you are not. They are allowed to stay out all night, but you are not. They are allowed to mingle with their ex, but you are not. They are allowed to lose or gain weight without judgment, but if you do, they will judge you for it. They are allowed to be lazy and do nothing, yet you are expected to be the one to do all the work around the house.

If you do not allow the narcissist to live out their free will, they will act out by getting upset with you. If you express your needs and desires, you will receive backlash from the narcissist. This is controlling and extremely unfair. Their evaluation of what is or isn't fair will not make sense to you or anyone else. Because the only purpose for their set of rules is to gain more compliance from you, the rules change constantly. Remember that they are only thinking about themselves and what will benefit them.

CHECK-IN

Take out your journal and write down ten things in the form of affirmations that you love about your character, such as "I am generous, I am kind, I treat people with respect, I always try to take care of the other person's feelings."

Now read all the points out loud. Now write down, "What gives my partner the right to feel they are more important than me and that the rules don't apply to them?" Answer this question for yourself and allow feelings of anger, disgust, or frustration to arise. Those are your friends—they are telling you that this hypocrisy is not okay!

12. they pretend to be a positive spirit while actually being a grinch

This tactic is constantly in use. They always seem like a positive bubbly spirit to the outside world, yet as soon as you are alone with them, the grinch inside them comes out. We already spoke about a similar tactic, when you are the only one who sees their true colors, but it can extend further than that. The narc will constantly burden you with their (negative) opinions of others, then smile in that person's face, pretending to be best friends, when they see them. They will burden you by complaining how horrible your family is, then plan fun golf weekends with your brother. They will pretend to love your pet and yet mistreat them. This can be an incredibly isolating experience. Everyone else views them as this loving, caring, sweet, charming person because they have perfected these masks, yet no one but you is exposed to their other side. Here are two examples to illustrate what I mean.

Example 1: Your partner is extremely entertaining, funny, and charming to every single one of your friends. They entertain the whole table by making jokes and being the center of attention. Everyone has a great night—or so you think. As soon as you're in the car leaving the restaurant, the mask falls off and all the care in the world about these people dissolves. Your narc complains about your idiot friends, criticizes the restaurant, and becomes someone who hates the world, especially you. You are left to deal with the uncomfortableness of the situation.

Example 2: You are at a parent-teacher conference at your son's school and the teacher explains your son's behavioral issues—he was yelling, and he bit his classmate. To your surprise, your narc wife responds calmly. She promises the teacher that the home environment is calm and loving, and she acts shocked to find out about the yelling, as "there is never any yelling at our house, and I don't know where he picked it up from." You know that this is untrue but say nothing. She further reassures that you'll both talk to him and make sure this never happens again. Once the meeting is over and you're in the car with your son and your narc, the switch happens: You're both stonewalled and not allowed to say a thing while she makes a speech about how stupid and incompetent this teacher is; no wonder your son is acting out. Once home, of course, she starts yelling and cursing at your son for being a nuisance and an embarrassing idiot who made her look bad in front of the teacher. She freaks out at how bad of a light this shines on her and starts yelling at you for being a crappy father and not raising your son better.

Another classic narcissistic behavior is constantly hijacking situations. Imagine you two are preparing to go to a family holiday dinner and your partner creates a huge drama, saying they don't want to go, criticizing your outfit, and devaluing your family right before you get into the car. The whole car ride is spent in silence and sadness. The narc's goal here is to put you off balance and make you feel upset, guilty, ugly—you name it. The scary thing is, despite just causing a fight with you and having a horrible car ride, the narc will put on their mask and act completely normal, with a smile on their face, at the holiday dinner with your family while you are trying to digest what just happened, knowing all the horrible things they have just said about your family. Even if you try to put on your own mask of smiles, your family will most likely sense that something is off. This will leave your family questioning why you're so upset or angry, and maybe your partner even cracks a joke or two on your behalf about how you woke up on the wrong side of the bed this morning, and all your family members laugh at it. Bless them; they don't know the half of it. You do.

This can be applied to any type of situation. Bottom line: The narcissist knows when they need to put on their masks and when they can take them off. As everything with them, it is calculated, and that is the dangerous part.

13. they use intermittent reinforcement

Intermittent reinforcement in a narcissistic relationship is when your partner displays their behaviors unpredictably. Love and hate are intertwined and inconsistently given to you by the narcissist, for no apparent reason. They go from being super sweet to extremely mean without any explanation. This unpredictable switch in behavior can feel like a complete change in personality; you experience your abuser like Dr. Jekyll and Mr. Hyde—one minute the sweetheart you love, and the next moment the monster you fear.

The narcissist is controlling the dynamic of the relationship by creating mini highs and extreme lows. You can visualize this dynamic as an unpredictable wavelike movement, with a constant back-and-forth between the narcissist giving you love and taking it away. When waves of affection come crashing in, they are strong and intense and create feelings of reassurance that the narcissist loves you. When the waves start pulling back, you are left bereft of all affection. The withdrawing drowns you with sadness, pain, and despair, leaving you struggling to regain your breath and hoping for a glimpse of joy, love, and attention once again.

This back-and-forth movement creates a trauma bond connecting you to your abuser. Trauma bonding is the strong emotional attachment between a survivor and their abuser. It is what I call a "chemical cocktail" addiction. The chemical cocktail you are addicted to stems from the love-bombing phase, which elicits serotonin, norepinephrine, dopamine, and oxytocin in your brain. Their charm-and-sweetness overload makes you feel on top of the world. *This cocktail is a dangerous combination of neurotransmitters and hope that no one is immune to. Do not blame yourself for falling for this drug. It's the strongest one that exists.*

Further, during the lows, the trauma bond has you desperately trying to reach your high again. You may begin to become obsessed with gaining back their love and affection on a regular basis, and this has you doing anything and everything for it. Just like an addict, you are willing to sacrifice your health for one more hit of their love. Being addicted to them leaves you begging for their affection, as you mistakenly believe they are the only one who could fill the void that you are now feeling inside. Every tiny piece of gentleness and care they throw at you seems like a huge deal now. The disturbing irony is that in reality you're receiving only breadcrumbs of love, but you've been conditioned to see them as gifts.

REMINDER:

If your partner is displaying hot-and-cold behaviors, do not continue to engage. This is a very toxic trait, as it can cost you your sense of self-worth. This is the essence of why you will start putting up with the abuse. It's the fundamental element of manipulation. You see those moments of their greatness, but actually it's the bare minimum, and you have been conditioned to be grateful for it. We will explore more about trauma bonding in chapter 4.

14. they make you walk on eggshells

A narcissist will constantly have you walking on eggshells. You may find yourself experiencing persistent tension all over your body. You never know when they will randomly explode again. Out of fear of retaliation, you likely do whatever it takes to keep them happy. Over time, you've become skilled in the art of hypervigilance, constantly monitoring their moods and reactions in order to avoid a fight. When there is something on your heart, something that is bothering you and you want to share it with your partner, you hesitate. You question whether your partner will be receptive to it, and nine times out of ten you sense that they will not be—so you remain silent. To keep the peace and stability of the relationship, you may avoid sharing your feelings altogether, especially if in the past your partner has threatened to break up with you. Time and time again, you consider what action of yours might create chaos in your partner and avoid those actions.

When you walk on eggshells, there is no room for healthy communication within the relationship. Since you will go to extreme lengths to keep or restore the peace, you will rarely get your emotional needs met.

I remember how I felt during one therapy session with Sage when she was talking about her experience with walking on eggshells. I could feel her fear running through my veins as she was describing the scene.

Sage's Story

"One night I was making dinner, and as I set the table, I froze for a moment. Should I give him Coke or Dr Pepper? Last time, he snapped at me for 'not knowing what he likes,' so I chose Coke, but I felt anxious the whole time, knowing he changes his preference on the daily. When he sat down, he ignored the drink but frowned at the plate and said, 'Why didn't you make the pasta the way I like it?' I knew I had followed the recipe he once said he loved, but I still apologized, telling myself it wasn't worth arguing over. After dinner, he was unusually quiet, scrolling through his phone. I felt the tension building and asked if he was okay, but I was so careful with my tone, terrified I'd set him off again."

When Sage found the courage to share specific details from her abuse, we were able to pinpoint how much instilled fear can be internalized. It was a life of constant anxiety trying to please her partner and be flawless. After several sessions of reflection, she was able to realize how much of herself she lost trying to anticipate his moods, apologizing for things that weren't her fault, and constantly questioning if she was the problem.

15. they say all their exes are crazy

This toxic trait should be an immediate red flag—when they claim that all their exes are crazy, something is wrong. As mentioned earlier in the book, it is not unusual to have an unhealthy or "crazy" ex-partner. This can happen to anyone. But when your partner says *all* of their exes are crazy or bipolar . . . *Ding! Ding! Ding!* Major red flag! If all their exes are crazy, what does that say about them? It either indicates they are a terrible judge of character when it comes to picking the right person, or they are simply lying. When someone says that all their exes are crazy, it also often means they have commitment issues.

Why does a narcissist do this? They discredit their exes to protect themselves. If an ex tries to warn you or spreads "bad rumors," or you hear anything positive about the ex, you're less likely to believe it. By priming you to see their exes as "crazy," the narcissist ensures you doubt any abuse stories that surface and instead view their exes as vindictive or unstable. This tactic gives them control over how you perceive the situation, no matter what happens, keeping you aligned with their version of reality. The last thing they want is for you and their exes to connect and expose them, so they manipulate your perception to prevent that.

16. they are unable to sit still

Narcissistic people have a hard time sitting still. They struggle with being alone, which leads them to constantly be on the go. Whether it's filling their schedule with friends or planning vacations one after the other, they physically find it hard to relax. It is not part of their nature. Why? Because they are constantly on the search for their next supply to "suck dry" for admiration, attention, and an ego boost. They can't give that to themselves.

The best way to spot this behavior is in a relaxing, calm setting where, despite the peaceful surroundings, the narc is unable to chill. Their behavior will come across as though they are on edge. Why is that? While you may be enjoying their company, it is not the same experience for the narcissist. They are in their head thinking of ways they can manipulate you to get more of what they want or need from you. I understand if this sounds morbid, but it's true. This sort of on-edge behavior can cause tension for you. You may not have realized it, but it's possible that you are feeling on edge as well when you are with them. Their behavior may also lead you to feel like you need to calm them down, entertain them, or prevent them from getting upset. This is exhausting, as you need to constantly be aware of their moods. Once again, their needs are being attended to in order to keep the peace.

Sharon's Story

"I had sold my soul to this man. I knew I had to go for good or I would lose my mind, end up an alcoholic—or worse, have a heart attack. I was so stressed all the time and had no peace. He never left me alone, and if I didn't do what he wanted, he would be passive-aggressive. I felt like I was in a cult."

Additionally, a narcissist is easily bored. They simply can't listen to a conversation that is not centered on them. They need to be the most important part of the conversation, and to ensure this happens, they actively insert themselves and make it all about them. For example, you share a story about being happy for a coworker who received a promotion, and instead of asking about which promotion they received or which coworker it is, the narcissist will talk about their own (often made-up) successes. Now suddenly the conversation is all about them, and the narc is fulfilled.

Moritz's Story

"I remember congratulating a coworker on her promotion one afternoon. I was genuinely happy for her—it was well deserved. Later I mentioned it to my girlfriend, expecting a simple 'That's great!' Instead, she started a monologue about her own 'big promotion' from years ago, one I'd never heard of before, though we'd been living together for years. She went on and on about how her success had been so impressive and how everyone was in awe of her. We no longer spoke about my coworker's accomplishment; it just became all about her. It wasn't even subtle; I was so over it at this point of our relationship that all I could do was roll my eyes and think to myself, 'It's just another moment where her need for attention takes over!'"

17. they try to engulf you completely

A narcissistic partner will do everything they can to engulf you completely in their life. From the moment they meet you, whether you notice it happening or not, they will try to get you to drop everything you have in your life—your friends, family, interests, hobbies, and so forth.

Through gradual manipulation and control they will carefully get you to drop each aspect of your life until they have you completely absorbed into theirs. Keep in mind that they are not interested in sharing *your* life. It is *their* world, and they want everyone and everything to revolve around it.

This is something that initially can feel wonderful. It can feed your own narcissistic needs of being seen, loved, and cared for—being the most precious person for the one you love. It's like you're all they need, and they are all you need. It gives you a "me and you against the world," Bonnie-and-Clyde, ride-or-die feeling that only the two of you matter and you don't need anyone else to be happy for the rest of your lives. You have found your soulmate. You are all each other needs. That engulfed feeling can feel magical, addictive, and wonderful.

However, this creates a codependence on the narcissistic partner. You no longer have your own life away from the relationship. There is no "us" either because all you do is live their life. As soon as they withdraw from your mini bubble, while you have left everyone else on the side (family, friends, and so on), you will be completely alone. Now you realize that there is no one left, that you are isolated, that you can only talk to their friends, that you can only spend time doing things that they love to do. This makes you feel lonely and vulnerable. With no world of your own, you are dependent on theirs.

This is a massive and damaging toxic trait. When the narcissist has engulfed you into their life, you are almost like their puppet; it's as if they completely own you. Your sense of independence and autonomy is taken away from you.

CHECK-IN

Think of your life in seven categories. In your journal, visualize them by either drawing them in pillars, boxes, or bubbles, then write them down as a list:

1. *Emotional (confidence, self-fulfillment)*

2. *Occupational (school, work)*

3. *Mental (art, entertainment, intellectual pursuits)*

4. *Financial (how you make and spend your money)*

5. *Social (friend groups, social activities, hobbies)*

6. *Physical (health and body appearance)*

7. *Spiritual (things that help you grow as a person)*

Now think of how your narc has managed to "hijack" some—or all—of these categories. Perhaps you quit your job to work for them, you changed your religion for them, or you no longer pursue your favorite hobby because the narc doesn't find it worthwhile. Go through each category and see whether your narc hasn't managed to overtake these areas of your life. Then look at that list or that drawing. Take it all in. Now make a promise to yourself that from today on, you will ensure that you do you and no longer do them, and you will fight back—even if you're still with them—so you can slowly start owning your life again. Take it step by step. It is okay to start small.

18. they cause you to feel constant anxiety

Experiencing nonstop anxiety when you are around your partner is a great indicator that you are in a relationship with the wrong person. Your narcissistic partner views their own needs and feelings as much more important than yours. Through their tactics and manipulations, they ensure that sooner or later you hold the same view, and you put them first. While temporarily putting your partner's needs first—such as when they're sick, grieving a loss, or losing a job—can be healthy, it becomes harmful when it's the rule rather than the exception. Having it be default can be draining and lead to anxiety, as you're nonstop trying to please them without listening to your own needs.

You are no longer living a worry-free life because they won't let you. If you forget about their well-being and don't put them first, even just for one minute, they will punish you for it. The constant stress of avoiding their punishment leads to catering to their needs more and more. This is the point where you are no longer focused on what you want for yourself, but you are now, at least partly, immersed in your new purpose: trying to fulfill their "Ten Commandments" at all times.

You're constantly trying to maintain peace and restore calm in your body, but your narcissistic partner won't let you. No matter how perfect you try to be, they thrive on chaos and drama. Boredom, for them, is intolerable. As a result, they keep you on edge, worrying whether they'll like your dinner proposal, fearing their moods when they come home, being scared that they'll leave you, or fearing that they're cheating. You're anxious about whether they'll show up to your child's play, humiliate you in front of others, or comment on your body, personality, or interests. The list of worries is endless, and it's gruesome.

At this point, your life revolves around minimizing pain and maximizing their happiness. You're constantly tiptoeing around them, trying to make them happy at the expense of your life energy. The toll this takes on you is not only physical but also emotional and mental. When your needs and desires are not being met, you may begin to feel anxious and depressed. A healthy relationship should never require you to perform constantly or fulfill your partner's every need. If you feel like you must constantly meet their demands, think twice about what kind of relationship you're in.

This constant pressure to keep their needs and desires satisfied can leave you feeling like it is never enough. For any narcissist, there is no such thing as "enough." A narcissist will never give you the reassurance that all you do for them exceeds their expectations or that they simply appreciate it. Why? *Because this is expected of you.* Therefore, when you are not receiving any thanks or appreciation hugs and kisses, it makes you wonder even more whether you are not doing enough, which only increases your anxiety.

CHECK-IN

If you are feeling like I hit the nail on the head with this last trait and you are experiencing more anxiety now, please make sure you jump to chapter 6 for a few minutes, where I show you in detail what breathing exercises and meditations you can use in this exact moment. These two- and three-minute breathing exercises and meditations will calm you, ground you, and give you a sense of inner peace.

---

19. they use your vulnerabilities against you

An especially cruel toxic trait is that the narcissist will use your vulnerabilities against you. In the beginning, when you share your insecurities, fears, or any type of vulnerability, the narcissist will appear empathetic. They will pretend to care about your vulnerabilities and interrogate you about them in a sweet way so that they find out every single detail about your traumas during the love-bombing phase. You will perceive this as true interest. Unfortunately, when the narcissist ends the love-bombing phase and enters the devaluing phase, they will attack. They will use every piece of information you provided against you, leaving you baffled and speechless with disappointment from the betrayal.

For instance, let's say you confided in your narcissistic partner about your strained relationship with your mother, sharing how difficult your childhood was and how little contact you have with her now because of how she treated you. When you have a random fight, out of nowhere the narc will use this painful information against you. They will say things such as, "No wonder your mother doesn't love you!" or "Your mother didn't treat you right because you're simply pathetic!" The narcissist does this to drive a stake into your soul. They know exactly what buttons they need to press to hit home and truly hurt your feelings. A classic tactic is using your body image against you. In the beginning they will tell you that you are gorgeous and perfect just the way you are. But sooner or later they will stop giving you these compliments and twist those once loving words into cruel ones.

No matter how the narcissist exploits your vulnerabilities, it will make you feel regretful for telling them in the first place. A partner should never make you feel bad about your insecurities, fears, or any type of vulnerability. They should support you instead and be your cheerleader when you don't believe in yourself. To spot this toxic trait in the beginning of a relationship, give them a fake vulnerability and see whether they will use it against you. #staytoxic.

20. they constantly ignore your boundaries

In the beginning, overstepping boundaries can come across as a sign of true romance. The first dimension of eroding boundaries is seemingly innocent romantic gestures—things you mostly experience during the love-bombing phase. For instance, if you have a busy schedule and communicate that you can't always text back right away, they will still shower you with texts or calls. This can seem sweet at first. You might think to yourself, "Look how much they are into me; I am always on their mind." You will feel flattered. They might drive you to and pick you up from every appointment you have, coincidentally show up at a party you told them you were going to with your friends, or basically live with you without having discussed it at all. You may view these boundary crossings as sweet and innocent at first, and they could be objectively seen as that—for now.

As the relationship continues, you go into the second dimension, which is the more intrusive and possibly even obsessive boundary-crossing phase. You might see that these oversteps are no longer cute, and they might start feeling uncomfortable, but you would still justify their behavior as passionate and romantic.

They might start doing things like answering your phone for you when you're in another room. They might use your computer to look up food deliveries while actually scrolling through your private folders—just to show you an old picture of you and tell you how cute you look in it. They could be texting you nonstop when you told them you have an important appointment, "just because they miss you so much" and start worrying when you don't reply. More invasive and even less cute are things like going through your mail and opening it while you're not home, reaching out to family and friends to make plans even though you're not in touch with them, or pretending to look for scissors on your desk while going through your drawers. In reality, all these examples count as clear red flags—a disregard for your boundaries.

Still, you're probably not going to say anything confrontational to them yet, as they always gaslight you into pretending what they're doing has a "sweet" intention, and you want to believe them. Let me show you an example by way of dialogue based on Sophie's story.

> **SOPHIE:** *Daniel, why is my journal out? Did you go through it?*

> **DANIEL:** *I did, but only because I care about you. I came across some things about your past—I had no idea you went through so much. I just wanted to understand you better so I can make sure I never hurt you like that. You deserve to be happy, and now I know what you need.*

> **SOPHIE:** *That's . . . really personal!*

> **DANIEL:** *I get that, but don't you see? I'm doing this for us. Knowing what you've been through means I can make sure I'm the person you need me to be. Don't you want that too?*

> **SOPHIE:** *Oh, um, I guess.*

What usually happens inside you is that you start to experience a strong ambivalence in these moments. For the first second when you witness these things, you might get a slight ick feeling and think to yourself, "Wow, this is a bit much. It makes me uncomfortable!" But only two seconds later you think, "Actually, this is really sweet. Maybe I'm being too critical. I need to start seeing the good in people, and they mean well." This is understandable but dangerous, as it will end up with you tolerating their BS.

You must admit, after reading Sophie's story and reflecting on your own examples, it is most likely no longer cute, but rather scary for you. You will begin to realize it is simply a way for the narcissist to keep tabs on you and increasingly invade your personal space.

Another dimension of eroding boundaries is by crossing sexual lines. When there is something specific (sexually speaking) you told them you don't like (e.g., bondage), they will start pressuring you about this topic more and more. They won't stop talking about it, brag how their ex did it with them, show you porn where it happens, and want to incorporate that exact thing in the bedroom "to loosen you up more." If you dare remind them that it turns you off, you're labeled as boring or a prude. They will make you feel bad by saying that you're such a baby, or they'll ask you why you're so closed-minded and unwilling to try something new. They might say, "You know that I enjoy doing X, Y, Z! You should finally try it for me." This leaves you feeling uncomfortable, unworthy, and not enough. You will feel pressured into complying with their needs more and more as time goes by.

Ironically, this also goes the other way, as you can't win with a narcissist. If you are (sexually) more open-minded than them, they will exploit you for it too. They will say things like, "That is so gross. I can't believe you would do something like that. I'm not sure if you are marriage material." They will make you feel dirty and inferior for it. The truth is, they are most likely envious of your adventures or jealous of who you learned it from.

No matter what boundaries you set, there is no winning with a narcissist. They will always make your boundary the problem. If anything, reasonable boundaries become even more of a challenge for them to destabilize. They don't play by any rules; they make them up as they go, so your boundaries mean nothing to them. They will never respect them, and you can never find "the sweet spot" by trying to set perfectly reasonable boundaries—it is purely wasted energy.

21. they never truly support you

A narcissistic partner will never truly support you. When you share any achievement with them, instead of celebrating your success, they respond with jealousy or another discrediting emotion. Rather than offering support, they diminish your accomplishment, making it seem small and downplaying its importance. They will also quickly turn the attention back to themselves by bringing up one of their own successes or achievements. This also becomes an opportunity for them to triangulate you with an ex-partner or someone they know you dislike.

For example, you might share that you received a raise at work. You'd expect your partner to be just as excited as you are. Instead, your partner downplays your accomplishment, saying it's just a small raise and not as significant as a promotion their opposite-sex "best friend" received. This hits even harder if you come from a family that also discredited your accomplishments, especially if your parents triangulated you with your sibling(s). Another reaction to your exciting news might be jealousy or frustration because they aren't getting a raise themselves. Either way, they will never admit they are doing this and will say you are paranoid if you call them out for it. The lack of support from your partner can make you feel as though you are never good enough in their eyes. This can leave you feeling isolated, unappreciated, worthless, and emotionally drained.

22. they want to control you in every aspect of your life

A narcissistic partner will feel the need to control your every move. As with everything a narcissist does, initially the sneaky control trait might seem sweet, as they will point out things they like. They'll tell you they love it when you wear conservative outfits, how you're most beautiful without makeup, how funny you are, how hot your chest hair is, or how sexy it is that you are so intelligent. At first the control appears in the form of compliments, but what you're not aware of yet is the flip side of that coin. That flip side sounds like "Don't you dare wear tight clothing," "You look stupid with makeup," "Can't you ever be serious?," "Don't you dare shave!," and "Don't you dare fail at your job." If you don't adhere to the implied suggestions, they will slowly start making your life difficult and blame you for the disharmony within the relationship. Their argument is "If you just comply, we have no issue," suggesting that if it weren't for your stubbornness, there would be no problems.

Naturally, when you're in love, you will try to fulfill your partner's wishes, even if they might seem a bit off to you. But remember, *no matter how much you try to cater to a narc, it will never be enough*. Their desire to control you and your life will exponentially grow, making it impossible to keep up with their requests as they become demands. The control will spread into and contaminate every aspect of your life. They will try to manage your social contacts (family and friends) by suggesting exactly who you're allowed to hang out with. They will start criticizing your appearance when you go to work and influence your ability to freely communicate with work colleagues or your boss. They will start triangulating or speaking poorly of others in order to have you doubt these people's worth in your life. They will ask you to stop surrounding yourself with people you highly value, such as your children, your parents, or your best friends. If you don't comply, at first they will act really sad and disappointed. If that's enough to keep you from seeing these people, great. If that doesn't cut it, they will get angry and create a scene. They will worsen the intensity of their dramatic tantrums until you withdraw from your social contacts in order to keep the peace at home. This is done out of pure manipulation. Their single goal here is to isolate you from everyone who is a threat to their sole control over you.

A quite dangerous part of controlling you is the financial aspect. A narcissist will lure you into creating a joint bank account. They trick you into believing that joint finances are a representation of a healthy, loving, trusting bond, when really they want to exploit you. Either you have more money than they do and they want full access to it to deplete you, or you have less money than they do and they see the perfect opportunity to trap you. Either way, their only aim here is to get full transparency of every move you make financially so that they can control that aspect of your life. The financial interrogation might start with questions like, "Is this membership really necessary?" then shift to demands like "Stop buying the kids lunch every day or else I'll limit your credit card."

More often than not, they literally steal your money and stash it away (and always have a great excuse ready) or spend it on ridiculous things, while keeping you on the shortest leash and complaining about grocery bills. In the worst-case scenario, they take all your money, leaving you with nothing or using that money to control you.

I have had many financially successful clients who lost their fortune due to their abuser. Their abuser forced them to take out unnecessary loans (that were often spent on affairs), cosign on business deals that went bust or were never even real, and swipe their credit cards for irresponsible purchases. In awful cases, these clients are now bankrupt with cosigned credit rates over their head that they are still paying off years after the breakup, forcing them to live at the bare minimum standard even though they have great sources of income.

Vivian's Story
"I discovered he'd been hiding money away, tens of thousands of euros, to spend on this other woman, while he complained that the pizza I ordered for the kids every Friday night was reckless spending."

23. they can't take any form of criticism

A narcissist is extremely sensitive to any form of criticism, as their precious ego can't handle it. When there is a perceived threat to their image or abilities, they will respond with aggression, anger, frustration, a tantrum, or any other hostile reaction. To protect their ego, they will disrespect you, put you down, and undermine your abilities. Standard critiques they can't handle revolve around giving them parenting advice, undermining their authority, questioning their decisions, criticizing immature behavior of their friends, mentioning an unhealthy habit of theirs, or disapproving of something their mother did.

For instance, imagine the two of you are in a car and your partner is driving too fast. You kindly ask them to slow down for safety reasons, but instead of listening, they speed up and start insulting you, saying things like, "Geez, you're so boring. You clearly don't trust me! I didn't know I was dating a grandma (or grandpa)!" or they may say, "You shouldn't be talking—you're a terrible driver! You can't even park without my help."

This type of reaction will shock you because it is disproportionate to what just happened. The narc manages to take something innocent and completely blow it out of proportion. These explosive reactions keep you from voicing any sort of criticism in the future and now have you thinking twice before saying something you would like to change.

24. they use belittling humor

Belittling humor is first disguised as funny little jokes. These jokes range from subtle remarks that sting to more obvious insults that truly burn. For instance, you mess up a calculation on a bill, and your partner says, "Oh, honey, you're so cute. You have never been good with numbers." That might sting for a second, but you'll think to yourself, "It's not a big deal for someone to innocently make fun of me. I do that too. It's nothing." You might think that it is like when a little boy makes fun of a girl he has a crush on. That's the first stage of belittling humor.

As the relationship progresses, the jokes get meaner, more degrading, and more personal. The jokes will never subside. The narc will use all your vulnerabilities and exploit them by constantly belittling you. At first it might just happen when the two of you are alone, but more often than not, belittling humor occurs in the presence of others. When others are there to witness your degradation, it hurts more deeply. Imagine you two are out for dinner with friends. At the dinner, your partner says in front of everyone, "Oh, babe, be sure to use a calculator for the tip! We don't want a repeat of when you overpaid the heating bill!" This is a classic example of exploiting and belittling you in front of an audience. It brings positive attention to them and negative attention to you as your intelligence is being undermined. Equally painful is when they belittle your looks, not your intelligence, as in this example:

YOU: *(reaching for another plate at the buffet)*

NARCISSIST: *(chuckling and speaking loudly) Whoa there! Save some for the rest of us! You're not trying to reenact Thanksgiving dinner, are you?*

YOU: *(frowning) I was just grabbing a little more. What's the big deal?*

NARCISSIST: *Relax! I'm just joking. But you do go for seconds like it's the last meal on Earth. We're in public, honey—might want to dial it back a bit.*

YOU: *That's not funny. It feels like you're making fun of me.*

NARCISSIST: *(laughing) Oh, come on, you're so sensitive! I'm just teasing you. You really can't take a joke, Miss Piggy?*

Over time, these little sarcastic jokes will build up to be horrible and crude comments. These are designed to make you feel worthless and small, as the narc has the most control over you when you feel like that. Your partner's humor shouldn't hurt your feelings.

keep notes to keep your sanity

If you have not done so already, document and save every form of toxic behavior and abuse your partner inflicts on you. Even if it's the smallest or "stupidest" little thing—anything that feels off to you, write it down. This can be done by taking screenshots of text messages, saving voice messages or voicemails, taking and saving video or audio recordings of your arguments or fights, having visual proof of physical abuse, or whatever you can use as proof of their abuse and lies. Something that I find extremely helpful is to create a section in your notes app on your phone and use it to write down all the bad moments with your narc. Make sure to put a date and time stamp on it as well. The more detailed, the better. This will help you when you decide to break up with or divorce your partner, as it will remind you of the long list of abuse. Trust me, if you don't write it down, you will forget, because stress and anxiety affect memory. If law enforcement gets involved, you will have concrete evidence of the abuse. This is simply a way to begin protecting yourself. As the brain is designed to repress the bad things and keep the good, this action of documenting all the bad will be a great reminder to you of all the horrible things the narcissist has done.

The bottom line: You are not crazy. You are caught in a trauma bond with a narcissist. This is truly a storm that you will need to navigate and is the focus of the next section.

part two

navigating the storm

chapter 4

trauma bonding

"Trauma is not what happens to you but what happens inside you."

—Dr. Gabor Maté

After reading through the damaging effects of narcissistic abuse, it is completely understandable to ask yourself, "Why did I stay for so long?" Whether you have found your personal answer to this question yet or not, please do not judge yourself for it. Hold some compassion in your heart. Regardless of your personal reason, there is a scientifically proven universal reason why people stay with their abusers. It is called trauma bonding, and it is a key consequence of all the tactics used against you by a narcissist. Trauma bonding is a very strong emotional attachment formed by you and your abuser, despite all the ongoing harm.

what is a trauma bond?

A trauma bond develops for three reasons. One reason is that your abuser alternated between love and kindness and cruelty and neglect, creating a confusing cycle of emotional highs and lows for you. Anytime your abuser showed love and kindness amid the abuse, your hope was reignited, encouraging you to stay (trapped) in the relationship. Trauma bonding is similar to Stockholm syndrome, the psychological tendency of a hostage to bond with, identify with, or sympathize with their captor. In trauma bonding, you form a positive emotional connection to your abuser as a survival mechanism. Due to this, rather than accepting the true nature of the abusive relationship and being forced to leave it, you develop a subconscious way to cope with the trauma that allows you to stay in it.

The second reason for trauma bond development is cognitive dissonance. You are stuck between facing the toxicity of the relationship and your awareness of your emotional attachment to the abuser. To overcome these conflicting realizations, you reduce your dissonance by focusing more on the positive aspects of the relationship and turning a blind eye to the obvious negative truths. You have most likely convinced yourself that if you keep being loyal and working even harder to do your very best, things will eventually return to how they were in the beginning (the love-bombing phase). That type of thinking further contributes to your inability to accept the reality of the abuse and break free of it.

I like to think of cognitive dissonance as a wave that you're trying to fight while stuck at sea, swimming as hard as you can, trying to survive and get your next breath. In general, as long you remain in the relationship with a narcissist, you will feel like this. You will be kept busy trying to struggle through everyday waves that come at you, trying to keep afloat, trying to swim through the stormy waters. You are so consumed with this fight that you can't see the shore. There is no way you can even think of giving up the struggle and swimming to safety. That's where the narc keeps you: occupied with their construed drama. That is, until you decide to do something to stop it and make your way to the shore. You can only do this by taking a deep breath and diving under the waves to get out of it safe and alive. Otherwise you will stay stuck in the narc-infested waters.

The third reason, and probably the strongest, is the chemical addiction in your brain that the narc has ignited. This is a more complicated process based on brain chemistry. The "chemical addiction" is your body's response to the emotional highs and lows (their intermittent reinforcement) of being with the narcissist. Your brain has come to expect—and crave—the stress that comes with alternating between conflict and resolution, tension and relief, that you are going through in your relationship.

Now that you know about the trauma bond, you need to understand the obstacles you will face in breaking its hold and getting free of the abuser. Remember, knowledge is power!

understanding the obstacles

The abuser's power seems omnipresent, and even with all this knowledge and education on the topic of narcissism, your heart still loves them. Even if your brain is telling you to run, your body is telling you they are worth fighting for. This is the trauma bond holding you in its grip. But once you understand the obstacles to breaking up with your narc and getting past your trauma bond, you'll know what you can do about them. Imagine each obstacle as a wave trying to pull you back to the stormy sea (your relationship, where you feel like you're constantly drowning) when all you want is to get safely to shore (a calm place where you no longer have to fight to survive). To do this, it is best not to fight *against* the pull but to work *with* it.

obstacle 1: what-if moments

What-if moments are very sneaky. They make you doubt your every move, past and present. These are the alleged "If I just hadn't done/said/thought XYZ, things would still be great between us" thoughts. You might be thinking things like:

> *If I hadn't gone through their phone, I never would have found out they lied. Then we wouldn't have had that huge fight where they stopped talking to me for a week and things would still be okay between us.*

> *If I didn't work so much, they wouldn't drink every single night. They told me that they need more of my attention. I have just been so busy trying to keep our finances in check.*

> *If I dressed sexier and had more of a sex drive, they wouldn't have cheated on me.*

Let's face the reality here: These thoughts are an aftermath of abuse, and your mind is playing massive tricks on you. Your abuser has forced you to feel as though everything is your fault, when the truth is they are the one that was in the wrong. *You have internalized the blame, and these are negative intrusive thoughts consuming your mind.* Even if you had not gone through their phone, they still lied.

The fight only happened because they were unable to take responsibility for lying, not because you found out. They drink too much because they have an attention and alcohol problem, not because you are working to help support the two of you. And it is their fault for not being able to stay loyal, not because you are not wild enough in the bedroom.

You can't take full responsibility for their actions. A healthy partner tells the truth and asks for your forgiveness if they've lied. A healthy partner communicates that they wish you worked less, or they would offer to work more themselves and take on the financial responsibility in a way for you to work less so the two of you can spend more time together. A healthy partner communicates their wish for more intimacy within the relationship and tries their best to make it more appealing for you.

CHECK-IN

Focus on the facts, not your what-if thoughts. In your journal, write down the facts:

1. *What happened? (They lied, they drank excessively, they cheated, etc.)*

2. *Who was in control of that action? (Answer: They were.)*

3. *Reframe the what-if thought. ("I am not responsible for their choices.")*

The bottom line is, you cannot carry the burden for two and bear all the responsibility. Of course, there are moments in a healthy relationship where one gives substantially more than the other—times of illness, the birth of a baby, the death of a loved one—but this is momentary, not a forever thing. It eventually balances itself out and neither of you should have the feeling that you carry the whole load. But when you are with a narc, you are the only one ever carrying anything. One partner carrying all the responsibility on their shoulders is *not* healthy, *not* normal, very toxic, and exactly what narcissists let you do.

obstacle 2: wishing on a star

We all know this one. It's another little cognitive dissonance trick. Your mind is set up very intelligently for survival. It tends to forget the bad and cling to the good in order to survive. This is a coping mechanism your brain automatically reverts to so you can function in your everyday life. If our brains did not do this, any bad event would manifest into trauma quite easily and haunt us, preventing us from moving on and living a happy and productive life.

Unfortunately, with toxic partners, this coping mechanism is counterproductive. When you are with a narcissist, clinging to the good makes you reinvest in the abuse cycle rather than stepping out of it! This is dangerous and not helpful. It is vital to understand that this healthy programming will not work in an unhealthy relationship. We all have it and appreciate it under regular circumstances, yet when dealing with a narc, it is vital to un-brainwash yourself from this deeply rooted programming and actively, consciously turn against it. You do not need to feed into this loop of suffering. Take a step back and see it for what it's worth. Just because they said or did something nice does *not* mean they will become a decent human being or anyone that you can have a healthy, loving relationship with. You can't rehabilitate a narcissist.

When the narcissist throws breadcrumbs of affection or attention toward you, you want to cling to them like they are the most amazing things, like lifelines. You will use their every "okay" move as proof of potential to be their sweet (manufactured, fake) old self again. Their intermittent reinforcement is fueling your hope for better times. Every single breadcrumb they feed you creates an out-of-proportion reaction of gratitude that adds to your big hope of them becoming kind and loving again. Here are some examples:

Look how gentle they are with the dog today. They would make such a great parent!

Oh my, how sweet. They brought me tea in the morning. Things will get good again, I feel it. Today will be a great day.

Wow, they answered my text right away, even though they are at work. This must mean they love me again and are no longer flirting with their colleague!

Your need to see their moves for what they are: entrapment. See what they do, *not* what they say; measure *not* by what they promise but what they show you with their actions, consistently.

The word *consistently* is key here. You will find that if you stop any "what they could potentially be like" thoughts and refocus on the current reality, they will seem much less amazing than you imagine. They will be a hollow, cold-hearted narcissist that you need to leave, not a potential partner you are building castles in the sky with. Everything else is merely a dreamy idea, a plan in your head, a wish upon a star. Your dream is essentially something that *could* happen, given your view on their potential, but it isn't likely to be grounded in reality, given their true self.

If you are honest with yourself, you might have poured more of your faith into your partner than you have ever poured into your own parents or friends or anything else that is important to you. That's not because the narc is so much more deserving than everyone else but rather the narc and their tactics are so evil that it needs something pure to balance it out. They have spread so much darkness in your life that you have made it your subconscious job to balance out the darkness by pouring all your light, faith, and love into them, hoping that they will see it, appreciate it, and one day return the favor. Subconsciously you want to save them from themselves and try to recreate the fairy tale you had in the beginning.

CHECK-IN

Write down two examples of where you put more faith into your narc than they deserved. This could be trusting them with something important, relying on them to organize something, or hoping they would behave in a way that would sit right with you, even if you weren't there to witness it.

obstacle 3: i will never find love like this

Your partner is the only person in the entire world who can so tangibly make you feel loved and worthy (when they want to)—all you crave is more of that. All you want is to get back to that first-weeks feeling where you were convinced that you'd found paradise with your "one." I get it—you feel you tasted the forbidden fruit and you don't want to let go of it now. Your craving for them is so strong that it feels like nothing in the world can help you change your mind. The only thing that satisfies this craving is being with them and waiting for their care (currently their breadcrumbs).

As I mentioned before, loving a narc is like being addicted to a class A narcotic such as heroin. *There is no stronger drug in the entire world than another human being.* In the beginning, your love is so intense and amazing, just like the intense euphoric feeling of the first hit. Most addicts spend the rest of their lives trying to get back to the feeling from their first hit. They waste away emotionally, mentally, and physically while chasing the dragon continuously. They are so involved in their chase that it often takes them years to realize how far off the path they are and how much they've lost along the way. Once they realize their addiction, it's a long, hard road to recovery. Only the lucky ones are able to recover; the unlucky ones literally die for their drug.

You have a choice.

Just like an addict, you can kill yourself trying to get back to paradise with your narc or you can get into recovery. In this moment, you most likely can't see what is going on, but you need to pause, breathe, and open your eyes. You need to understand that no matter what you do, you will never again get back to lasting paradise with them. Your paradise was never real. It was what they wanted you to see. It was all manufactured to get you to this desperate place you're in now. Believing harder in them than in yourself is wasting your life, your aspirations, and your dreams—wasting it all on them.

Recognize that by refusing to let go of your illusions, you are keeping yourself trapped in their abuse cycle. Decide now to confront the situation as it truly is, no matter how difficult, and take responsibility for freeing yourself from the fairy tale that's holding you back.

obstacle 4: denial

Denial is a mechanism that exists to avoid painful truths. It is fundamental in any toxic relationship. It has to be there by definition; otherwise, toxic relationships would cease to exist past a couple of weeks because the first red flag would create an unease so big that you would walk away.

More often than not, denial starts right at the beginning of a narc abuse relationship and unfortunately lasts way past the breakup. In the beginning, you will be in denial by minimizing the abuse and downplaying everything your partner does wrong. This results in later excusing their inexcusable behaviors. To justify their behavior, you might think, "They are only so controlling because their ex cheated on them!" Excusing their faults goes hand in hand with the next part of denial: pretending everything is okay when it is not. But these are mechanisms to "protect" your relationship and your abuser from the judgment of the outside world. The outside world isn't wearing your rose-colored denial glasses. *If you told your truth, it would become real. The abuse would become real. So, you don't.* This leads to self-blame, where instead of blaming your abuser, you blame yourself for protecting them.

Another part of denial is avoidance behaviors, which can manifest in different forms. A classic example is self-medicating in order to "function." This is done so you can push aside the obvious truth that the relationship is not healthy and you need to leave. Many abuse victims have tried minor tranquilizers (Valium, Ativan, Xanax) to cope with the stress of abuse. They need to feel sedated enough to stop the anxiety that gets in the way of caring for children, working, and managing household chores. Some try sleeping pills to get through their nights calmly. The problem is that these medications are highly addictive, and you will need more and more in order to get the same effect. *The fact that you have to self-medicate to endure your partner's treatment should serve as a wake-up call that something is really wrong.* No one should need drugs just to handle their relationship. This is a huge red flag.

Please stop all of it. Don't further protect your abuser in any way, shape, or form while hurting yourself.

CHECK-IN

In which aspects exactly are you protecting your abuser by denying the truth of their behavior?

---

obstacle 5: fear of judgment

Fear of judgment manifests in three specific ways when dealing with narc abuse. First and foremost, you are constantly worried about being judged by your narcissistic partner, as what matters most to you is what they think of you. If you ever tried confronting any of their wrongdoing, they would quickly turn it back on you and judge all your past behaviors and attack your character. You are not wrong to be worried about this, but you need to start seeing through them. One of my friends, Dr. Sara Al Madani, says, "In order for someone to be able to hurt you, you must first value their opinion." Take that to heart. Why would you value an evil person's opinion? Why would someone's construed reality that you know is not true get to you so much? Why would you choose to believe their gaslighting? It is time to face the reality of your abusive relationship and stop allowing their words to have any weight on your self-worth.

Second, you are worried about being judged by everyone else about your perfect relationship that isn't so perfect after all. In the beginning, you spoke so highly of your partner that you might think no one would believe you if you now changed your story 180 degrees and said that this nice person is actually abusing you. You might think that if you now speak poorly about the person you protected for so long, others will think you're making it up. You know that all they have seen and heard is the nice, charming side of your partner, and it worries you to death. You think, "I used to do everything in my power to keep this picture-perfect image, and now I'm smashing it. Of course they will judge me."

Even if all that were true, there is no better time than now to break the illusion. If you don't act now, things will only get worse. The sooner you act, the better.

It is important to pause here and take a breath. Just because you have these thoughts does not mean others will too. The ManKind Initiative, citing the UK's 2022–23 Office of National Statistics, reports that one in seven men (13.9 percent) and one in four women (27 percent) will be a victim of domestic abuse in their lifetime. Therefore, many people will relate to what happened to you. Don't forget that these figures are likely much higher because, just like you might have, people keep abuse a secret. If you speak up with your truth, you might be surprised by how you may help someone else find the inner strength to voice their abuse too. Even if some people judge you, the good you can do—not only for yourself by sharing your story but also by giving others courage—is worth far more than the "silly" opinions of some very small-minded people. Remember, your partner has groomed you into believing that if you say anything bad about the relationship, you are the bad person; the narc has convinced you that no one will believe you, and you will be seen as the crazy one. This is simply not true.

Last but not least, the third fear of judgment is the most painful. It is realizing that the harshest judge of them all might just be *you*. It means coming to terms with the fact that you voluntarily got involved with a narcissist, voluntarily ignored the red flags, and voluntarily continued to keep the relationship afloat despite the abuse. Realizing that you lied to protect your abuser and still chose to wear your rose-colored glasses is very painful. It may lead you to doubt and at times even hate yourself. Rather than have compassion for yourself, often all that's left is self hate and shame—shame and hate about your failed sense of character, your inability to judge situations, and your skewed perception of others.

> ### CHECK-IN
>
> *Imagine it's not you; it's your best friend suffering your story. How would you react? Would you judge them and make them feel bad for it? No. You would hold immense compassion and understanding. You would hold their pain until they calmed down. You would let them feel all their feelings and tell them it's okay. You'd hug them and hold them. That is what you need from yourself now—patience, kindness, and compassion, not judgment. Turn off your inner critic by telling them to shut up for once, and be your own best friend.*

It's okay to fear the possibility of judgment for a moment. Just take the next moment to face that exact fear and fight it with your knowledge. You know better than fearing judgment. You know the truth. You have lived the truth. You have endured the abuse. You were the victim once, but with the right mindset, you are now a survivor.

obstacle 6: dependency

If you are with a narcissist, you likely feel very dependent on them for everything in your life. If they have a bad day, you do too. If they choose to be nice, you feel grateful and relieved. Even in a healthy relationship, this is normal to a degree, as you always want things to be smooth and your partner to be happy. But abusive people really take advantage of this codependence. They aim to create it and blow it up. They do this in several ways.

The narc has emotionally manipulated you into becoming dependent on their validation. They did this through repeatedly making you feel incredible in the beginning, as though you were their one and only. You never felt as special as you did then. That feeling is addictive and gorgeous, and everyone wants more of it, naturally. The problem is, in time, they started slowly making you feel all sorts of ugly emotions: guilt, shame, fear, belittlement, judgment, and insecurity. After all the praise, these new emotions confuse you, as they make you feel weak and small. You desperately want to get back to the beauty of the beginning, so when they finally give you praise or words of affirmation (breadcrumbs of love), you thrive! You think, "Finally, they are kind to me again! I have to do more of XYZ behavior so they continue to be so sweet."

This grooming is already happening. These "praises" are often minimal and mostly only words, no action. But like breadcrumbs to a starving person, you are so grateful for the praise and want to believe them. You cling to every nice word, as their opinion means so much to you. This is when they have you in their pocket. A narcissist is an expert controller and manipulator. The sweet words and empty promises in between serve only them. It makes leaving them much harder, as you are experiencing the intermittent reinforcement we spoke about earlier.

This emotional dependency also further exacerbates fear of isolation. Over time, the narc has you isolated from your previous sources of love and support. All that is left is them. There is no one around now to validate you emotionally, except the narc. The narc is often your sole emotional anchor, your entire world. There is no one else around to tell you the truth. At this point, your self-worth and self-esteem are relying purely on them. This is extremely dangerous, as they intentionally use it against you to keep you feeling small and worthless. They have inflicted this self-doubt so much that you actually feel lucky to be their partner and are frightened to death to be without them. Just the thought of being without them causes serious anxiety in your body. You feel so unsettled and scared that you start acting in strange, psychologically fragile ways. You obsessively check for texts from them. You find yourself impulsively lashing out, then regretting it. You start tantrums where you're crying on the bathroom floor. You start fights for no reason and later feel ashamed of your behavior.

Basically, you're being extremely insecure and acting neurotic, which they never miss to point out and make you feel horrible for. Your narcissistic partner will ask, "Why are you so clingy? Why are you so jealous? Why are you being such a baby?" The answer: It's them driving you there. They gain an omnipresent power over you.

But remember, *a person can only gain as much control over you as you give them*. Even if you are emotionally and financially dependent on your partner, you have no reason to allow them this much power. There is always a way out, which we will get to later.

Let's touch upon financial dependency. You might be confused about how this happened, especially if you were financially independent, even doing well for yourself, before meeting your narcissistic partner. Unfortunately, the narcissist has likely found a way to take control of your finances. They may have convinced you that a joint bank account was the best option for you or the family, or persuaded you that they were better suited to manage the finances or family business and should have access to all the money. In more extreme cases, they may have manipulated you into signing documents that cost you your savings or led to bankruptcy. Sometimes the narcissist was the sole provider from the beginning, reassuring you that you didn't need to worry and that they would take care of everything—especially your children. This was perhaps something you craved so much that you were willing to look past the red flags. Don't blame yourself; it is also understandable. You came from a place of longing, and they fulfilled that dream of someone taking care of you, and you thought you found your perfect savior.

Regardless of how it happened, the narcissist has gained control over your finances, creating one of the most devastating forms of dependency—financial dependence. Now they hold complete control over you financially, leaving you feeling powerless. You may find yourself asking, "How can I leave if they control all the money?" or "How can I save when they have access to all the bank accounts?" It might feel like staying is the only option. But don't let the weight of this reality stop you from exploring your options or taking action. *You always have a choice*. You are not trapped. The prison inside your head.

We have just explored some of the many games your brain can play on you when you have formed a trauma bond with a narcissist. But it goes deeper: The trauma bond and the abuse cycle with a narcissist can lead to some very severe mental health disorders for you, and this is the subject of the next chapter.

chapter 5

how narcissistic abuse affects you

"Narcissistic people don't want unconditional love.
They want unconditional tolerance."

—Unknown

Realizing and accepting that you are with a narcissist can feel scary and painful. For so long you have been catering to their needs, chasing their love and affection, and playing damage control, all just to keep the relationship afloat. But what about you? What is happening to you throughout all of this?

After recognizing and understanding the abuse cycle and tactics narcissists use against you, it is vital not to underestimate the effects their abuse will have on your mental health. The five phases of the narcissistic abuse cycle cost you not only your psychological and physical strength but also your spirit, demoralizing you to the point of complete devastation. This devastation leaves scars that often accompany you for a lifetime, leaving you to internalize all their blame and making you feel worthless. This worthlessness is instilled by experiencing any type of abuse over time, something I've seen quite often in my clients.

Each type of abuse is heartbreaking, but there is one common symptom that summarizes the effects of narcissistic abuse: *difficulty or even inability to make any sort of rational decisions because you are so stripped of your self-efficacy and no longer able to trust your own instincts or intuition.*

As a professional therapist accompanying many clients through their darkest times of abuse and post-abuse, I find self-doubt to be the most dangerous consequence of all, considering its massive detrimental effects. If you can't trust yourself, you can trust no one. You lose your trust in anything and everything. Without any sense of trust—in yourself, in others, and in your life—recovering and moving on is extremely difficult.

mental health conditions as a result of narcissistic abuse

During and following an intimate relationship with a narcissist, the most common serious mental health conditions that occur in survivors are post-traumatic stress disorder, complex post-traumatic stress disorder, and narcissistic victim syndrome. Let me give you a short introduction to all three.

post-traumatic stress disorder (PTSD)

In worldwide literature, you will read that narcissistic relationships cause post-traumatic stress disorder (PTSD). Although this was once widely accepted, more recent findings indicate that narcissistic abuse survivors often don't suffer from simple PTSD but rather complex post-traumatic stress disorder (C-PTSD). I would still like to explain PTSD in a few words, in order for you to understand the difference.

PTSD is an anxiety disorder that develops when you are exposed to a one-off, short-term traumatic event. If you suffer from PTSD, you will have symptoms of intrusion (distressing memories, flashbacks, or nightmares), avoidance (deliberately staying clear of reminders of the trauma to avoid re-traumatization at any cost), random mood changes, and hypervigilance (constant heightened state). PTSD brings a sense of helplessness and sometimes even personality changes. You could be experiencing all these symptoms and still suffer from C-PTSD, as I will now explain.

complex post-traumatic stress disorder (C-PTSD)

C-PTSD is a form of PTSD and may appear similar, yet it is crucial to make a distinction between the two. The major difference is that *C-PTSD carries elements of captivity, loss of self-worth and identity, and a continual tendency to be revictimized.* Losing your sense of self contributes to the severity and complexity of this disorder, hence adding "complex" to the diagnosis. All these elements do *not* exist in simple PTSD.

C-PTSD is a complex form of PTSD that develops when you are *continually* exposed to traumatic events, such as being in an abusive narcissistic relationship. The following six symptoms can help you recognize whether you are suffering from C-PTSD:

1. **Changes in mood regulation and impulse control.** You may start to notice emotional instability, such feelings of sadness that just won't go away, anger you can't seem to express, or even dark thoughts about self-harm or suicide. As these feelings begin to take over, it becomes harder to control your reactions, and emotions feel overwhelming.

2. **Changes in attention and consciousness.** You might find yourself disconnecting from reality, dissociating from the present moment. Instead of being able to focus on reality, you are stuck reliving intrusive memories or flashbacks that remind you of your traumatic experiences.

3. **Changes in self-perception.** You might begin to perceive yourself differently, typically in a more negative way. Often, feelings of helplessness, shame, and guilt take over. You may even feel paralyzed by self-blame and self-hatred for what has happened because you start to believe the abuse is somehow—or fully—your fault.

4. **Changes in relationships with others.** At this point, you are so scared of your abuser's immense power over you. It feels like they are omnipresent in controlling your life. Yet you might find yourself defending them in front of others, as you are still caught in your trauma bond. As a result, isolation and mistrust of others grow stronger, which can make relationships with anyone but your abuser feel unsafe.

5. **Changes in physical symptoms.** Over time, your emotional pain turns physical. You may begin having panic attacks, anxiety, hair loss, fluctuating weight, gastritis, rashes, UTIs or other genital infections, and other physical symptoms. If you haven't already, you may have even sought medical help, hoping to treat the physical symptom, but nothing helped. The truth is the origin is not physical but rather rooted in emotional suffering.

6. **Changes in worldview.** Throughout time, your entire worldview begins to shift. Feelings of hopelessness and despair take over, and it becomes harder to believe in the existence of any future outside of your relationship with your abuser.

The psychological effects of C-PTSD are complex and will destroy your healthy sense of self. This is because when you are involved in an intimate relationship with a narcissist, they are your most significant attachment figure and thus have the most influence over your self-esteem. The emotional pain of enduring these C-PTSD symptoms will most likely lead you to question whether you're fundamentally flawed. This will eventually cause you to lose trust in yourself and your ability to make decisions. The constant self-doubt and insecurity can spill over to future relationships, where you risk being victimized again.

narcissistic victim syndrome (NVS)

A special form of C-PTSD in connection to a narcissistic abuse relationship is called narcissistic abuse syndrome or narcissistic victim syndrome (NVS), which is marked by severe deficits in self-confidence and mental health caused by living with a narcissistic partner. This syndrome is not officially recognized as a medical diagnosis but that does not take away the seriousness of it.

The psychological effects of narc abuse are profound and can be long-lasting. The narcissist's relentless manipulation and abuse strip away your sense of self and worth. You are trapped in a constant cycle of cognitive dissonance, questioning your reality and struggling to trust yourself and others. During the relationship, and often long after it ends, you may feel a deep, permanent sense of isolation. Shame becomes overwhelming, leading to self-sabotaging behaviors as you internalize the abuse and blame yourself for it. This can result in self-harm and even thoughts of suicide.

The intensity of this psychological damage can make it difficult to function in daily life, start new intimate relationships, and reclaim your autonomy. NVS is the devastating result of the abuser systematically attacking and destroying the very core of who you are. The following list can help you recognize whether you are suffering from NVS during and/or after a breakup from a narcissist.

1. **You feel like the relationship was absolutely perfect in the beginning.** Abuse typically begins very slowly, after a very strong love-bombing phase in the beginning.

2. **You feel like you constantly have to walk on eggshells around them.** You try to avoid another drama by doing anything and everything to keep your partner from having an outburst. You are constantly careful about what you say and do, since anything can spark a narcissist to lose control.

3. **You feel isolated, vulnerable, and alone.** The isolation causes you to doubt your perception of situations and rationalize the abuse. It's easier for the narcissist to manipulate you when you feel you have no one left to turn to. You might even feel that the abuser is the only one you have.

4. **You have a pervasive sense of mistrust and paranoia.** You may feel especially anxious and hypervigilant when it comes to anyone who represents a slight threat to your sense of safety.

5. **You engage in self-sabotaging behavior.** You replay the abuse in your head over and over again, ruminating on what you could have done differently. This fuels negative self-talk, self-blame, and self-sabotage. You may begin to self-harm, engage in other self-destructive behaviors, or become suicidal. The abuser increases their power by putting you down, and as the chronic abuse continues, you may begin to punish yourself for enduring the toxicity, developing something known as "toxic shame." Over time, you may stop pursuing personal goals, feeding into your sense of worthlessness. Often, you're already isolated from friends and family, leaving you without anyone to offer an objective perspective or remind you of your worth.

6. **You experience unexplainable physical symptoms.** Your immune system must work much harder when cortisol levels are at a constant high. This leaves you susceptible to illness and physical weakness; insomnia, fatigue, changes in appetite, stomachaches, ulcers, constant migraines, muscle aches, and panic attacks are very common. These physical symptoms, known as psychosomatic symptoms, can't be explained organically.

7. **You struggle to put up any boundaries for yourself.** Abusers generally leave you with little sense of respecting boundaries, as every time you tried to set one in the past, you were severely punished or humiliated. The silent treatment and mind games mess with your head, making you question your sanity. Even in future relationships, you might struggle to set healthy boundaries as you've learned that your boundaries were repeatedly disregarded in the past. Leaving an abuser requires putting up strong boundaries, which we'll explore later.

8. **You question your own identity.** Your abuser constantly makes you adjust your beliefs to their every desire and need. You experience moments where you feel detached and dissociated from yourself. This happens because the abuse is so overwhelming that your mind tries to cope by splitting off fragments of yourself.

9. **You find it nearly impossible to make decisions due to a lack of self-esteem and self-confidence.** During chronic narcissistic abuse, the narc makes you believe that you are unable to make any good decisions or survive without their help and insight into life. After a while, you start to believe these instilled thoughts and make them your own. Their gaslighting makes you doubt yourself over and over again, which leaves you feeling insecure about whether they are right and you are worthless and useless.

10. **You are the object of a smear campaign created by your partner.**
Sometimes, after a breakup, people take sides and support one party or the other. Particularly after narcissistic abuse, the narcissist will do anything in their power to get your friends' and family's support to make you feel alone. This can cause severe distress and depression, provoking the feeling of having no support network, even perhaps losing the closest people around you and feeling completely isolated.

CHECK-IN

It's very common to see yourself in these descriptions and blame yourself for staying with your abuser. Instead, imagine yourself as a five-year-old who tells you that they really messed up in kindergarten: They stole the class teddy bear and took it home. It looked so pretty and felt so cozy, and they just wanted to play with it alone. Your little self feels really horrible and shameful for not telling the truth when the teacher asked. How would you treat your little self? Would you blame them, scream at them, and criticize them? Or would you hug them and tell them, "It's okay! You can't change your past, but from now on you can do better and bring it back"? I hope you would choose option B. Now, as an adult who "messed up" by staying with a narc longer than necessary, please do the same. Hug yourself and be understanding and loving instead of shaming yourself further. You cannot change the past; you can only control the present and therefore change your future. Once you realize how much time you spent trying to deny reality, decide to get help, and then with that help, walk away now and never look back.

Now that you have a clearer understanding of how narcissists can affect you, and you understand some of the mental health conditions they can cause, it is time to focus on how you can manage their impact.

chapter 6

coping tools during the relationship

"Do not let the behavior of others destroy your inner peace."

—The Dalai Lama

T here are many things you can do to manage the stress and difficult feelings you experience while dealing with a narcissist. This chapter includes my favorite techniques and interventions that have helped my clients over the years. I suggest you try these and see which ones resonate the most with you. Keep in mind that timing is very important and, often, exercises don't feel good one day but feel great the next. It's about being ready and open to surrender to these exercises, and that can be especially hard during times of heightened anxiety. Some of these might work best once you're out of the relationship. You can try them again later if they don't do their magic for you yet.

therapy and connection

"I was able to see that it's okay to not be okay."

—Michael Phelps

I know I am biased, but you have to trust me when I say therapy is an essential pick-me-up when you are constantly fighting a battle of survival. Don't try to be a hero and do it yourself. The statistics are against you. You need some form of therapy to find your strength again and help you focus on your goal: breaking free of your narc.

Go online and find a therapist in your area who specializes in any one or more of the following therapies and try them out! It is an individual experience, and you never know which ones will work for you, so be open to surprises. Once you find a great trauma therapist that you vibe with, stick with them and try to do a weekly or biweekly therapy session for some months. I promise, good therapy with someone you connect with will change your outlook on life quite quickly. Remember that working on yourself benefits not only you but also everyone around you, whether that's your children, siblings, parents, friends, or work colleagues—everyone benefits from a better version of you. The only one not benefiting from a stronger version of you is your narc—and that is exactly what you want: you regaining power. I recommend the following types of therapy most often to my clients.

animal-assisted therapy

"Until one has loved an animal, a part of one's soul remains unawakened."

—Anatole France

Animal-assisted therapy (AAT) is magical. Animals hold unique abilities to heal through their unconditional love and nonjudgmental presence, something rarely seen in humans. The things I have seen happen in clients through animal interventions are astounding. I have seen children who are nonspeaking speak for the first time in years when they worked with snails. I have seen people finally open up about their fifty-year-old secret when they were hugging my horses. I have seen clients truly understand that their pain is seen and validated when Amari, my dog, licked their entire face and sat with them until they downregulated themselves during a very intense trauma session.

Science has documented many benefits of AAT. Since animals offer unconditional love and empathy, they create feelings of trust and acceptance in AAT clients. Research shows how this bond is transformative, especially for people suffering from trauma and (C-)PTSD. The human-animal bond reduces depression and loneliness while increasing feelings of self-worth and empathy. As a therapist working with animals, I find AAT the quickest way to get straight to the heart. It simply moves mountains if done right and leaves the client with a heart full of love and a huge smile on their face. The results are astounding, much better than those of only talk therapy. If you like animals at all, you should seek out AAT near you and give it a try.

> **CHECK-IN**
>
> *In your journal, write down a short reflection exercise on your favorite animal.*
>
> 1. *What is it about this animal that makes you feel connected to it? Gentleness? Loyalty? Strength?*
>
> 2. *How does thinking about this animal make you feel?*
>
> 3. *If you had this animal with you during hard times, what comfort might it offer you?*
>
> 4. *Imagine how its presence could even change the way you handled a difficult moment.*
>
> *Think about how you can incorporate these qualities into your healing journey. Perhaps seek out AAT? Spend more time with pets? Volunteer at a local shelter? Google your local options!*

trauma therapy

"The greatest discovery of my generation is that a human being can alter his life by altering his attitudes."

—William James

There are many therapeutic modalities that address specific traumas. The most well-known trauma therapies are cognitive behavioral therapy (CBT), mindfulness-based stress reduction (MBSR), mindfulness-based emotional processing (MBEP), eye movement desensitization and reprocessing (EMDR), and brainspotting.

COGNITIVE BEHAVIORAL THERAPY (CBT)

CBT is a widely used evidence-based approach that can help C-PTSD through reframing your negative thought patterns. It is considered the top-notch treatment for trauma. The model states that our thoughts, feelings, and behaviors are interconnected, and through changing the negative spin on our thoughts, we can also change our emotions and behaviors. It is a highly structured approach and typically short term, as it focuses on specific goals such as healing the emotional abuse you went through.

MINDFULNESS-BASED STRESS REDUCTION (MBSR)

MBSR is an eight-week program that incorporates mindful meditation to help you increase awareness of being present in the moment. By focusing on the body without judgment, you are able to create a nonreactive awareness of thoughts and feelings associated with your trauma. MBSR decreases activation of the brain's fear center while strengthening the brain's decision-making functions. This modality is very effective in fighting negative ruminations that usually follow after being romantically involved with a narcissist.

MINDFULNESS-BASED EMOTIONAL PROCESSING (MBEP)

MBEP is one of my favorite trauma therapies, and I use it a lot for deep trauma with my clients. It raises your awareness of the trauma stored in your body and helps you process the emotions associated with them without being overwhelmed. This can be particularly helpful after traumatic experiences with narcissists.

EYE MOVEMENT DESENSITIZATION AND REPROCESSING (EMDR)

EMDR helps reduce the emotional impact of distressing memories through bilateral stimulation, or alternately stimulating the right and left sides of the brain. This can be done through guided eye movements while you focus on traumatic memories of your narc. It shifts your memories from the limbic system, which is responsible for emotional responses, to the prefrontal cortex, the area of the brain responsible for planning, decision-making, and self-control. Therefore, traumatic memories become easier to process logically, and the brain can store the memories without the same emotional intensity. It is very well known for reducing C-PTSD symptoms quicker than talk therapy.

BRAINSPOTTING

Brainspotting is a fairly new trauma therapy based on the premise that where you look (the brainspot) affects how you feel. Brainspotting works by identifying specific eye positions that correlate with unprocessed trauma stored in the brain. During therapy, you are asked to focus on a specific spot in your visual field while simultaneously focusing on traumatic memories. The brainspot taps into your body's natural ability to heal, particularly accessing deeper brain structures where trauma is often stored. By holding the focus on the brainspot, you are able to process unresolved issues more efficiently than with traditional talk therapy, thereby reducing trauma symptoms. Brainspotting differs from EMDR by emphasizing the stillness of the gaze rather than bilateral movement.

mindfulness, meditation, and breathwork

"Deep breathing is our nervous system's love language."

—Dr. Lauren Fogel Mersy

When you feel stressed, insecure, sad, anxious, depressed, or experience any other negative emotion that brings on intrusive thoughts, I suggest practicing mindfulness, meditation, and breathwork, which train your mind to stay present and keep you from dwelling on drama. These practices break cycles of overthinking, self-doubt, and hypervigilance caused by narcissistic abuse. They help you observe your thoughts without becoming emotionally snared by them. They also allow you to create mental distance from your abuser and recognize that your thoughts, often shaped by the narcissist, are not a reflection of your true self. I like to think of all three types of interventions as a way of resetting your focus back on yourself, after all you've done lately to focus on the narc. This gives you an opportunity to practice self-care in a beautiful, connected way.

Mindfulness and meditation help reduce anxiety and regulate your emotions. Mindfulness teaches you to stay present, guiding your mind and body out of the heightened state caused by the narcissist. Meditation provides a safe space to observe and manage your emotions, preventing reactions to the abuser's manipulations and triggers.

Physically, mindfulness and meditation offer you a refuge. By calming your body, lowering your blood pressure, slowing your heart rate, and enhancing your sleep quality, meditation will help you reduce the massive stress caused by the narcissist. When you're experiencing restless nights or battling insomnia, your mind becomes more susceptible to unhealthy, looping thoughts, further decreasing your well-being. By working against this and regaining peaceful sleep, you strengthen your body and mind, breaking the cycle of distress.

The Zen teacher Shunryu Suzuki Roshi, once said, "If our minds are like wild horses, we must give them wide pasture." I love this saying because it refers to anxiety as wild horses instead of something negative. This is a great reframe because it is true: All you need to do is create space for your horse (your mind) to be able to be wild (by meditating and breathing) without bothering anyone (creating anxiety). Following are some of my favorite techniques that you can try when you are feeling like anxious and need some space in your head. There are also countless breathing, meditation, and mindfulness exercises available free online and for purchase. I suggest downloading apps such as Insight Timer or Calm. They provide quick access to breathing, meditation, and mindfulness exercises.

DISCLAIMER

Some intense breathwork and meditation techniques are not advised while pregnant. I made sure to pick pregnancy-safe exercises for this book. If you are unsure of any suggested techniques you find on the internet, please check with your doctor before trying them. Also, for anyone suffering from mental illness, including temporary states such as PTSD, NVS, or C-PTSD, please double-check with your psychiatrist, as some exercises are not safe to practice if you are at risk for psychosis.

seated mindfulness

Here is an exercise you can complete in one minute to ground you during anxious times. It helps you focus on the present moment instead of stressful thoughts and feelings.

1. Sit up straight but comfortably, and have your feet flat on the ground.

2. Place your hands on your knees, and close your eyes.

3. For one minute, just focus on your breathing. Having random thoughts is to be expected, so if you have any, let them in, accept them, and let them go.

4. When the one minute is up, slowly open your eyes and continue with your day.

body scan meditation

A body scan meditation allows you to slow down, become aware of physical sensations within your body, and release tension. Here is a one-to-two-minute body scan meditation.

1. Find a comfortable position either sitting or lying down. Close your eyes, and place your hands in your lap.

2. Slowly inhale deeply through your nose, and slowly exhale through your mouth, allowing your body to relax.

3. Bring your attention to your toes. Try to notice any sensations, tension, or feelings of relaxation. Then gradually bring your attention to other parts of your body. Slowly work your way up your body, shifting your focus to your feet, ankles, calves, and so on, all the way up to the top of your head. Pause at each body part and notice the sensations you are feeling.

4. As you notice any tension or tightness in your body, breathe deeply into that area. When you exhale, imagine the tension leaving your body. That tension can be a color, a movement, or a symbol. Just imagine it as best as you can leaving your body.

5. Take one last deep breath. When you are ready, slowly open your eyes and resume your day.

break up with narcissism

R.A.I.N. of self-compassion meditation

The meditation teacher Tara Brach created the R.A.I.N. of self-compassion meditation for moments when you're stuck in feelings of unworthiness and insecurity. All you have to do is sit with your feelings and follow these four steps. This can be done in your mind or in your journal.

R ecognize what is happening.
A llow the experience to be present, just as it is.
I nvestigate the situation with interest and care.
N urture yourself with self-compassion.

For example, say you've just had an argument with your narc. They twisted your words, blamed you for something you didn't do, and made you feel inadequate for expressing your feelings. Now you're left feeling emotionally drained, angry, and questioning your own worth. Here's how to use the R.A.I.N. technique:

RECOGNIZE WHAT IS HAPPENING.

- Pause and name your emotions: "I feel hurt, angry, and confused. I'm questioning my own actions and wondering whether I'm at fault."

- Acknowledge the situation: "This argument was unfair, and I was made to feel like the problem."

ALLOW THE EXPERIENCE TO BE PRESENT, JUST AS IT IS.

- Resist the urge to suppress your feelings or rationalize the narcissist's behavior. Instead, give yourself permission to sit with your emotions: "It's okay to feel this way. These feelings are valid."

INVESTIGATE THE SITUATION WITH INTEREST AND CARE.

- Gently explore your thoughts and feelings: "Why do I feel so unworthy right now? Is it because I've been told my needs don't matter? Or because I've been made to doubt myself?"

- Reflect on the reality of the situation: "Does their reaction reflect who I am, or is this part of their pattern of manipulation?"

NURTURE YOURSELF WITH SELF-COMPASSION.

- Reassure yourself: "I'm not unworthy. Their words are not the truth about me."

- Offer kindness to yourself: "This is a hard moment, but I deserve love and care. I will treat myself with the kindness they don't."

- Engage in a comforting action, such as journaling your thoughts, drinking tea, or listening to calming music.

By applying R.A.I.N., you've shifted the focus from their hurtful behavior to understanding and soothing yourself. This practice helps rebuild your emotional strength and reminds you that their manipulation does not define your worth. Over time, this process empowers you to trust your feelings and break free from self-doubt.

alternate nostril breathing

Alternate nostril breathing is a yoga-based technique in which you breathe through one nostril while holding the other shut, then change nostrils and repeat the process. Research on this breathwork exercise has been found that after only one month of alternate nostril breathing, people showed better oxygen flow in their bodies, healthier lungs, and better airflow to the brain, which helps with clearer thinking. Try to do around five minutes of this exercise several times a week to get the most benefits.

1. Exhale through your mouth, making a soft *whoosh* sound.

2. Lift your right hand and use your thumb to close your right nostril. Inhale through your left nostril.

3. Close your left nostril with your index finger so both nostrils are now blocked.

4. Hold your breath for a moment with both nostrils closed.

5. Release your thumb to unblock your right nostril and exhale.

6. Pause briefly after exhaling.

7. Keeping your left nostril closed, inhale through your right nostril.

8. Close your right nostril again with your thumb, hold your breath for a moment, then release your left nostril and exhale.

belly breathing

Belly breathing, known as diaphragmatic breathing, is a technique that helps reduce anxiety and stress and improves breathing efficiency. Ideally, five to ten minutes of this exercise is great, but continue this cycle of breathing for as long as you need. When you notice that you have shallow breathing caused by your anxiety, belly breathing is the best way to deepen that breath consciously and help you calm down. Do this daily for the best benefits.

1. Find a comfortable position by sitting or lying down; your back should be straight.

2. Place one hand on your chest and one hand on your belly.

3. Inhale slowly and deeply through your nose. Allow your belly to rise as you inhale deeper; focus on the hand on your belly rising. The hand on your chest should not rise; it is there to be an indicator whether you are inhaling into your diaphragm correctly.

4. Exhale slowly through your mouth. Feel the hand on your belly lower as you let your breath out.

box breathing

Box breathing, also known as square breathing, is used by the US Navy SEALS as a quick way to get the nervous system under control. It helps you stay focused as you return your body to homeostasis after a stressful experience. If your body was in fight-or-flight mode, box breathing helps recenter yourself and improves concentration.

There are four basic steps, each lasts the same number of seconds (usually four). Imagine you are breathing along the sides of a square, and repeat for as many times as is comfortable for you. The goal is to focus on the rhythm of your breathing to reduce anxiety and stress and activate your parasympathetic nervous system to induce relaxation. Research suggests that, ideally, it takes about four minutes until your inner calm returns. Practice daily.

1. Sit up straight in a chair, with your feet flat on the ground and your hands resting in your lap.

2. Slowly breathe in through your nose and count to four. Make sure to fill your lungs fully so that your chest and belly expand.

3. Gently hold your breath for a count of four.

4. Slowly exhale through your mouth and count to four. Let out all the air.

5. Repeat for at least one minute.

4-7-8 breathing

The 4-7-8 breathing technique is also known as the "natural tranquilizer for the nervous system." It consists of breathing in for four seconds, holding the breath for seven seconds, and exhaling for eight seconds. This breathing pattern reduces anxiety and is especially useful for falling asleep, as you exhale double the time you inhale. It also lowers blood pressure and increases concentration. It takes less than two minutes, and you can do it anywhere.

1. Find a comfortable place to sit with your back straight.

2. Place your tongue against the back of your top teeth and keep it there.

3. Close your lips and inhale through your nose for a count of four.

4. Hold your breath for a count of seven.

5. Exhale completely through your mouth, making a *whoosh* sound, for a count of eight.

6. This completes one cycle. Repeat for three more cycles.

exercise

"Take care of your body. It's the only place you have to live."

—Jim Rohn

You don't have to be an athlete to reap the benefits of physical activity. Exercise is a natural way to relieve stress, reduce anxiety, and release endorphins—your body's "feel-good" chemicals. When endorphins are released, they help boost your mood and reduce feelings of pain, which can be especially helpful when dealing with the constant emotional manipulation, abuse, and neglect from your narcissistic partner.

The constant walking on eggshells, hypervigilance, and worry can build up tension in your body, and physical activity helps release this tension in a healthy way. Whether you walk, run, or lift weights, *you will feel better*. Even if you're not in the mood at the time, try to push yourself anyway—you will be glad you did. Consider joining workout classes such as Zumba, or a team sport such as volleyball, or a partner sport such as tennis. These are all great ways to stay active and get those happy hormones pumping, and they also help you regain some positive social connections. You might make important friends. This will help you build up your self-worth and decrease feelings of isolation. If your partner forbids you from joining a gym or signing up for a class—don't tell them! I don't like to suggest lying, but in this case, omission is for your own benefit.

setting boundaries

"'No' is a complete sentence."

—Anne Lamott

I know I've mentioned boundaries many times and told you that the narc will always disregard them, but it is essential that you try to establish and uphold them anyway. These boundaries are not just for the relationship with the narc but also a form of self-care and self-protection for you.

Do not allow your partner to cause further turmoil in your life. Begin setting healthy boundaries by saying no when you need to, and do not let feelings of guilt or obligation stop you from saying no. Resistance is to be expected. The narc will get upset because they are not used to hearing the word *no* from you. They feel they have lost control over you the moment you say it, because you have been so compliant in the past. They're not used to that! By saying no, you are beginning to take back your space and your power. "No" is one of the most powerful boundaries you can set while still in a relationship with a narc. Each time you practice saying it, you prepare yourself for the breakup. Learning to say no *now* will strengthen you for when it's time to break away completely, the subject of the next section.

part three

breaking free

chapter 7

escaping from your hell

"You must make a decision that you are going to move on. It won't happen automatically. You will have to rise up and say, 'I don't care how hard this is, I don't care how disappointed I am, I'm not going to let this get the best of me. I'm moving on with my life.'"

—Joel Osteen

It is easy to feel like all the narc's absurd pursuit of power over you has things spiraling out of your control. The coping tools in chapter 6 can help you calm down and get centered, but maybe you do not feel equipped enough for the full war that is about to unfold. It is important to try to keep your cool here and know that just because you feel you have lost all agency doesn't mean that it is true. Your narcissistic partner's manipulations and games have you in an emotional state, but this is not your truth. It's just a feeling. The key to actually breaking free of the invisible chains that are holding you back is understanding what is and what isn't in your own control. You can break free from the narc, and now I will show you how.

what is and isn't in your control

First of all, the bad news is that *you can never control the narcissist*. Even if you feel you have found a way to manipulate them, you will never win. You can't control their words, actions, or feelings, let alone the toxic energy they feed on. The more you get invested, the deeper you're pulled into their world and the more disconnected you are from yourself. Hoping for change while being with them is wasted energy, like trying to heal while on drugs. The contamination is a constant unwanted chaperone on your journey, and no amount of effort will decontaminate your surroundings until you remove yourself from its source—the narcissist.

The good news is, even though you can't control them, *you can learn to control yourself*. You can control your reactions and the power you give the narc. Every time you pause and don't react, you withdraw your energy and yourself from them. When you decide to stop playing their games, you get your energy back to use on yourself! That is exactly when healing can begin. Reacting less, giving them less attention, less focus, and less of your precious time is key.

This is simple, but not easy. The truth is, as long as you keep the narcissist in your life, your life will be contaminated. Even if you are no longer living with them but still in touch, the contamination lingers. Don't fool yourself: There is no alternative to this truth. You can't fix them. You can't change them. But it's in your hands to decide when to stop feeding their power and start reclaiming your own.

big decisions

I advise you to hold off with any big decision you are contemplating. It is vital to understand that abuse and trauma lead to mental confusion, therefore making any big decisions right now can be a mistake. It is best to allow time to pass, as you stabilize yourself and weigh all your options, before engaging in life-changing decisions. Also, you are most likely suffering from C-PTSD/NVS symptoms, which have your impulses all over the place. Making an impulsive big decision in the near future can have detrimental effects, as you might seriously regret it tomorrow, or next week. Do not make any pivotal decisions on career choices (quitting, starting something new, starting over), relocating (moving to a new city or even country), financial investments (taking out a loan, making risky investments), health changes (getting surgery, opting out of medical insurance, stopping therapy), education (deciding to enroll in or withdraw from a program), or family arrangements (divorcing the narc, marrying the narc, having another baby with the narc, adopting a baby). All of these are major life changes and should be decided with a clear, sober, strong head.

I am not saying that these decisions are not right or might even be perfect for you. Rather, I'm urging you to take a bit of time to make sure that you are in a decent headspace to weigh the pros and cons and really think things through. Of course, I encourage any decision that supports leaving your abuser, but it is important to note that if you are making a decision on an impulse, that same impulse may have you right back with your abuser a short while later, aggravating the situation. The key is less drama and less stress, and that is only attained by maintaining a cool, calculating head. You need to be ready to leave (for good) because there are many obstacles that come in the aftermath that you need to be ready for. So, making sure you are aligned with your decision is vital. Finish this book first. You do not want to put yourself in the position of having to undo a messy, impulsive breakup. It will only put more on your plate.

Whatever decision you are dying to make right now, mark one month from now in your calendar. If you still feel like it's the right decision then, and you haven't changed your mind more than once in between, go ahead. A great marker to cross-check if your decision is "good" is telling your closest trustees (not your abuser) and seeing what they think about it. Only tell people who will 100 percent support your decision to leave the narc (no mother-in-law, no jealous friend, no one who will talk you out of it for their benefit or bias).

Once you have made the decision to leave, it's time to make a plan.

preparing to leave

As with any well-thought-out plan, to leave an abusive relationship, you must prepare correctly in order to increase your chances of succeeding.

write it down

As we have already discussed, it's vital to have a list of all the moments they showed their true colors. This list is more than the ordinary "bad trait" list—it is a list of every single moment of "What was *that*?" in your relationship. It's best to start this list as soon as weird things begin to happen; even if you think it's just a tiny red flag, write it down. However, if you didn't start a list before, do it now. You will be surprised at the intensity it has once you reread it and revisit all the emotions you had while these things happened. The list might start out with small, unimportant events that just irritated you (for example, your narcissistic partner started a fight over something supermundane while watching TV on the couch) but can reach massively disturbing occurrences (for example, they tortured your dog while you were at work). It is so important to keep this list safely stored away from their eyes. Remember program syncs, such as iPad/computers/iCloud connections, and make sure the narc never finds your list. Always keep it close—ideally in a notes app that is *not* synced with other devices, hidden on your phone.

Another way to shore up your inner strength is a hate list. A hate list is just what it's called: a list where you write down all the things you hate about your narcissistic partner. This is just as important to create! It might seem like toxic advice from me to do this, but as soon as you are in the midst of leaving them, you will understand why. They use all their charm to try to lure you back, and it is really hard to resist them. If you have these lists, you can refer to them as your "safeguard from naivete." They will lead you right back into knowing how messed up the narc truly is and remind you of their faults. This will help you not cave into a fantasy of hope and, instead, stick with reality.

get your finances in order

The next step is to get your money in order. Whether you are broke and dependent on your partner or well-off and have nothing to worry about—or like most of us, somewhere in the middle—doesn't matter. You need to plan ahead financially whenever you break up with a narc. Financial intelligence is important regardless of the precautions you need to take. You may need to open a second bank account under your name, get a new job, get a loan, ask someone to cosign something for you, or get a lawyer who can help you protect your wealth. This needs to be thought through and executed before you have "the talk." Doing this after will be a mess, as they will try to control you through financial threats and ultimatums.

If you have shared assets, you must be especially clever. Get them to sell something or have them sign it over without letting them sense your plan. Depending on which state you live in and whether you are married, there may be "no-fault divorce," or you may need to prove to a court that you have been abused. Please seek out legal advice and find local legal services. Often these are free of charge and funded for victims of abuse. This book is not enough to cover those aspects, depending on your situation. The more information and support you have, the better prepared you will be for the breakup.

dealing with children

If you share children with the narcissist, or if the narcissist acts as a parental figure to your children (even if the children are not biologically theirs), my most important advice prebreakup is to make sure they are safe. This means ensuring that they are somewhere other than the location you choose to have your breakup in (more on that later). Whether that is in a café, your house, or somewhere else, your kids need to be away from the scene and the aftermath of it, not just in another room. The narc can't be able to reach them during their impulsive reaction time. This is the only way to protect them. No matter what age, witnessing a toxic breakup is extremely traumatizing and should be avoided at all costs. For them to simply see the effects it has on you afterward is traumatizing enough. Put them first.

getting help from the outside

I understand how isolated and lonely this whole relationship has made you feel. You do not need to continue to do this alone. In fact, I advise against it. As you prepare for the breakup, reach out to friends and family you trust to support you unconditionally. Often at this point in time, the narc has managed to completely isolate you from your support system, but there is always a way back. Real loved ones never fully turn their back on you, even if you have ignored them for months or years. They will often surprisingly take you back with open arms. There are also groups you can attend or online communities you can join for extra support, which will make you feel much less alone. It will show you how many other people are going through similar experiences and will help you feel connected to others. They can help you emotionally, as well as give you advice and guidance from their experiences. In today's world, we are quite lucky to be able to connect with others online so easily. Use this as an opportunity to help yourself.

Here are two websites I find helpful to connect to others going through the same thing:

Circlesup.com is ranked number one in narcissist relationship and divorce group support online. They offer weekly online group sessions.

Psychopathfree.com is a website that offers the opportunity to join online forums that relate to survivors of psychopaths, narcissists, and sociopaths.

Just like there are trusted people you *should* go to, there are also people who you *shouldn't* go to. Do not go to someone who is not entirely and unconditionally on your side. Only seek out people who will strengthen your decision to leave the relationship. You need biased helpers now—biased for your side of the story. No empathy for the narc, please. Do not contact their parents hoping for help. Do not contact their friends or family members, no matter how close you were before. They will most likely defend the narc and notify them of your intention to break up with them. Only stick with people who truly have your back.

organizing your physical move

In the difficult case of living together, you need to start organizing your move now. Find a new home, whether it is temporary (for example, with your parents, a friend, or a shelter) or permanent, if you have the capacity. Make sure your new place is far away from your partner, not in close proximity—unless you have shared children, then make it manageably far away. Also, if you live with someone other than the narc, make sure they will never tell the narc where you are.

Next, pick the day you will break up, and organize your move accordingly. Especially if you are a procrastinator, having a schedule will force you to go through with your plan and will leave no excuses open. This is one of the hardest parts of ending your relationship. It feels so final. And hopefully for you, it is. It helps if you're angry rather than purely sad—use your hate lists for this! Look at each of those points, each time they made you feel absolutely worthless, and get angry! Since you have already started telling your trusted people about what is going on, ask them for help for your big day. If you have the money, get some quotes from a moving company and organize your moving date. Obviously do this carefully so your narcissistic partner will not find receipts, emails, and such about your plan.

Make sure you organize your actual move when your narcissistic partner is not at home—ideally at work or out of town. If your partner is jobless, on your moving day you need to bring in the cavalry. Have your closest family and friends there so your partner can't intimidate you or keep you from leaving. If you are completely alone with this, try to get creative and gift your partner an activity they love to do for the day (golf day with friends, pub day with their bestie, hiking, spa day), and do it then.

Ruth's Story

"Knowing that if I engaged with my ex about separation/divorce it would not end well, I planned my exit strategically and without letting him know. He came home one evening to a letter I left for him. I had moved into an apartment while he was at work that day. He was blindsided. He was stunned. He absolutely thought I had left him for someone else. I did. I left for me. He blamed me. He was angry. He tried to coerce me into returning and giving him yet another chance. No. Not happening. Eight years later I have zero regrets."

You may be thinking, "I don't have anyone in the world who will help me. How do you expect me to leave?" But remember, this is not casually swapping houses; this is an airplane crash. You are not going to bring your favorite dinner table out of the psychopath's house. Forget material belongings. You are a survivor, and you will earn this name. All you need is *one* suitcase of your most important essentials and you are out of there. If you have kids, pack one backpack each. That's it. The rest will come later once you reorganize your life. Any place is better than sharing a place with your narc. You can do this.

You may be feeling inspired or absolutely overwhelmed. Both of those are equally okay. If you now have an action plan, I'm glad I fueled your fire! Keep going strong! If you are feeling overwhelmed, just pause the book here and take a couple of days to let it sink in. Take it one step at a time, at your speed, without impulsive decisions.

have a safety plan

Having a solid safety plan in place is absolutely essential, as leaving a narcissist can more often than not turn out to be quite dangerous. Prioritizing your (and your children's) well-being is the most important thing in the world. Here are some steps to follow *before* executing your plan.

1. **Secure important documents.** Make sure you have copies of or access to essential documents like your ID, passport, social security card, birth certificates (for yourself and your children), medical records, and financial information. Store these in a safe place or, even better, leave them with someone you truly trust.

2. **Pack an emergency bag.** In addition to your essentials in a suitcase or backpack, pack an emergency bag with basic clothing, necessary medication, a burner phone, and some cash to get you through the first phase. Leave this bag with a trusted friend, at work, or in another secure location outside your house.

3. **Have a code word with allies.** Create a code word or phrase you can use with friends or family to let them know you are in danger or ready to leave. For example, saying, "I'm picking up that blue sweater you like" could signal them that you are about to execute your plan tonight.

4. **Use technology carefully.** Narcissists often track you via your devices. If you suspect your phone or email is being monitored, use a different device if possible. Definitely disable all of your location sharing on your phone, and check privacy settings on apps and social media accounts.

5. **Trust your instincts.** Your intuition is your greatest ally now, even if you doubt it sometimes. If something doesn't feel safe or right, listen to that feeling and adjust your plans accordingly.

Remember, this is about your safety and survival, not about being polite, fair, or accommodating. You are your top priority, and no one else has the right to jeopardize your life or well-being.

putting your plan into action

Once you have your plan in place, you still need to execute it. The following suggestions will help make sure things go as smoothly as possible and you remain safe, as leaving them is the most dangerous phase in the relationship with an abuser. Especially if they abused you physically, you need to take extra precaution here.

pick a neutral place

A typical breakup usually takes place in a private setting away from others to see and hear. A breakup with a narcissist needs to be treated differently because it is important to de-escalate their reaction. Pick a neutral public space where you feel comfortable—and they don't. This ensures that they refrain from overreacting and escalating the situation because they don't want witnesses to their extreme behavior. I call this a preventative action to increase your success when breaking up with them.

CHECK-IN

You are probably full of sadness, guilt, and confusion right now, and all your heart wants is to mend the situation. I understand that fully, and I know the pain of a narc breakup is very different from a typical one. I am sure you would love nothing more than to have a sweet heart-to-heart talk in your living room where you explain yourself and get a loving and empathetic reaction from them, but this is an illusion with a narc. They will not react "normally." They won't respect your decision, hug you, and walk away in peace—they will try anything and everything to regain control over the situation. This is why it is so important to pick a neutral place where you can step away anytime and stay in control.

---

be a diplomat

First, limit your own emotional investment. To do this, you have to be ready to face the consequences of losing them. If you're not, keep working on gearing up the strength until you are. If you are ready, limit any emotional investment during your breakup talk to the bare minimum. This means that no matter what emotion comes up and what urge they trigger inside you during your talk (urge to mend, explain, understand, be sad, scream), try not to react at all and do not show them what is happening inside of you. You need to act as robotic as you can so you don't give them an opportunity to exploit your vulnerability. They will jump at any chance to entangle you.

Second, during this talk, it is not important to show your feelings and your personality; it is important to be stoic and smart. This talk is not about being authentic but rather getting rid of them. That is the only goal. Here it is actually advisable to take all the blame in a friendly demeanor. Keep away from aggressive behavior and tone of voice, and try to be calm and subdued. This is not a tip to make you cave but rather to de-escalate their response. You want to keep them as docile as possible. If you give them a reason to become more defensive (criticizing them, yelling), things will get out of control. Save your authenticity for supportive family and friends or your therapist.

Third, if you are afraid of not getting your points across without them interrupting your thought process, write down your reasons for why you want to break up with them on ChatGPT and ask Chat to write you a short, friendly, and precise breakup letter including all your points without any emotions. If you are not able to do this on your own, get support from ChatGPT or a therapist. Use it and read the writing out loud to your soon-to-be-ex. The key thing here is to keep it *short and clear*. A paragraph is truly enough, but the shorter, the better. The best thing you can say to a narc is "I don't love you anymore," as that is a blow to their ego and you have the best chance of them feeling hurt enough to be okay with separating.

In case the narc acts like a narc and does something such as ripping your letter up and saying, "Don't be stupid, baby, we belong together!," have a backup plan (and print two copies). You will not be thrown off guard as all you need to remember is one thing: a one-sentence reason you have on repeat. *This sentence is your lifeline and you will remember it by heart.* I will give you some examples that are clear and suitable for a narc. Of course, you can put it in your own words, but keep it short, concise, and, most importantly, something they can't argue away easily. I am telling you, they will try!

Here are some sample sentences to learn by heart and repeat like a broken record until you walk out on them:

"I am simply not happy with you anymore. It's over."
"I don't feel respected or valued, and I know I deserve more. We're done."
"I don't love you anymore. It's over."
"I am not interested in being with you anymore. We are done."

CHECK-IN

You will have the urge to explain all your feelings and pour out the truth and might even have the hope in the back of your mind that they will understand, promise to change, and things will go "back to happy" for a while. You need to ignore this hope. Even though hope is a beautiful thing, with an abusive partner, it is a useless thing. The chance of a narc changing themselves is 0.01 percent. It's not going to get better. So, if your hope is bigger than your conviction that you need to break up, don't do it yet. You need more time. (And that's okay!) If you are convinced and ready, make sure you keep to that one sentence after saying what you need to say and simply do not let them entangle you in further talk. Their solemn purpose now is to "win." Winning for them does not mean being happy with you but gaining the upper hand of the breakup situation. Either they want to keep you from breaking up so they can do it in two days, or they want to torture you further because they haven't found a better supply yet. Please be smart here. Let your brain take over by accepting that this will hurt, but it's the right thing to do.

say what you need to say and leave

This is quite straightforward, and seemingly easy, but hard to implement. Let's face it, you have a letter to read out loud, a speech you have thought through, and one sentence to convey on repeat. That should not take you longer than fifteen minutes, tops. Any time you leave open after that gives your narc a chance to drag you into a conversation that you no longer should want to take part in (as there is absolutely no point). Whether they will use the time to tell you everything you have been wanting to hear for years or they will use it to make you feel horrible, you can skip it because it has no benefit for you. These tactics aim to make you doubt yourself and your decision. Be wise. Don't let that happen. Give yourself a maximum of fifteen minutes with them, and don't allow any discussions to take place. Tell them you don't want to argue, and repeat your sentence like a broken record. Do not say anything else or engage with anything they say. Anything they say will be manipulations and empty words—nothing else. Don't give the narc one moment to interact with them. Leave them ignored like they used to do to you. When you are done, leave.

CHECK-IN

In a typical breakup, both partners may reflect on all the good and bad times spent together, giving each other a sense of closure. With a narc, you will never get closure. All you will get is lies, empty words, or manipulation to make you feel horrible and ruin any self-worth left. By eliminating any chance of a "possible resolution," you also eliminate their chance of manipulating you. You will not get a resolution, true closure, or the real apology that your heart so desires. You won't be able to feel that warm connection of friendship or true care for one another that you might feel in a healthy breakup. This is not only painful and disappointing but also frustrating, and it evokes feelings of unfairness. It isn't fair, but you can't fix it. Please don't try. You will not make history here and have a narc suddenly change their ways.

have an exit strategy

You now know that you need to keep it short and sweet. A well-planned exit strategy will help you do that. Ideally you need to enlist a trusted friend or family member who will be strategically waiting for you during this talk. Whether you're in a dog park or a restaurant, your friend can sit somewhere close by, where they can watch for your preplanned cues (raising your hand, throwing the salt on the floor in the restaurant—whatever your cue is) that you need help and it's time to leave. If they can't see you directly, have them on standby to reinforce your exit strategy as soon as they get a text from you. This ally should have a strong personality and not be intimated by your partner. If you are not able to have someone come with you, then make sure you have your own transportation home without the narc. They can't be in the same car, on the same train, or walking in the same direction when you leave the neutral meeting place. Instead, schedule a taxi or a ride-share pickup.

> ### CHECK-IN
>
> *The two hardest parts of a breakup: when you say you're breaking up with them—that's the easier one; and when you're actually walking away. Walking away can feel impossible. In that moment you might feel frozen, and your body doesn't want to move. You can't bear the thought of your next step because your mind knows that if you take that step, this is it. It's truly over. This is the final goodbye and your heart can't take the pain. Again, here you have to overrule your heart with your mind and just push through. Your heart will understand later that you were right in doing so. It's like jet lag. Your heart might need a few more days or weeks to get to the place your brain is at, but it will catch up with you. Let me send you all my strength now to have the power to walk away immediately when you're in that situation. And when you do, just know that I am so proud of you.*

protect your safety

If there is a risk of possible violent reactions (you know best), do not meet with your narcissistic partner to deliver news of your breakup; rather, do it over the phone or via an email without personal contact. If you are worried about your safety at all, please file a restraining order. You might feel like a coward for not "properly" breaking up with someone you loved so dearly, face to face. That's understandable, but special situations need special handling. Your safety is priority, not your pride in doing things "right." Protecting yourself is a courageous act, and you don't need to make it harder for yourself than it already is.

have your aftermath support ready to rumble

As mentioned in the previous section, make sure your trusted friend or family member is there for you after your breakup. It is important to have a plan for yourself. Ideally, after the breakup, you will meet different people in the evenings, spend time doing things you've been wanting to do, try out new activities. So, before the breakup, reach out to a support system, whether that's old friends or family you have, or new ones you try to connect with via online forums or other ways as mentioned and tell them what you are about to do. Have your calendar filled with a different person or activity (you can do so many things by yourself or with your kids alone!) every night so you are not feeling alone and not leaning too hard on one person. You have full permission to distract yourself and go to new places, as long as there is no chance of bumping into your ex. *Do not go to their favorite places or mutual friend events.* Do not interact with anyone who is even remotely on their side of the argument; disengage with everyone connected to your ex. If you love time by yourself, that is fine, but ensure that you will not be alone. Have a go-to ally or support hotline on speed dial, ready 24/7 to call if you feel like caving and going back to your ex. You need the support now, so please don't be too proud to use it.

Even if you feel like you have no one to turn to in your real life, remember that you are never truly alone. It's common to feel isolated when people around you seem preoccupied with their own lives. You might feel that you're not important to them or you can't reestablish a proper connection. However, there are numerous online communities and support groups that focus on exactly what you are going through where you can connect with people who have faced similar experiences with a narc. In fact, strangers online can sometimes become your strongest allies because they go about it in a different way than family or friends do. They might be able to help you out more, share their wisdom and success stories, and inspire you on a whole other level. Also, you can always see a therapist specialized in trauma and abuse. If therapy seems financially out of reach for you, explore pro bono options offered by some therapists.

Remember, for the duration of your relationship, the narc has made you feel as though you are not important enough or do not deserve support from others. Do not let those untrue, cruel words sink into your soul where you begin to believe them. Now is not the time to feel like you are a burden. Know that you are worth the support and love from people, and it is okay to lean on others for their help right now. This is especially tricky for people who are used to independently functioning in everyday life without relying on others for help. This is not a time to shine and be strong; this is a time to let yourself seek help and advice—not only because you need it but also to rewire your brain into knowing that most people are kind, empathetic, and generous, and you deserve all of that. Not everyone is toxic. You need to feel the love in order to outgrow the fear.

prepare for all the masks of deflection

As you already know, the game is always different with a narc, and that also goes for the endgame. They will not accept or respect your decision and treat the breakup like a healthy partner would. They will use all their manipulation tactics to get their control back. They may choose the "nice" way—that is, disguise their manipulations as attempts to solve your issues and pretend to understand; they may even say they will change and get help. All of that is fake.

Do not fall for it. Or they may choose the "mean" way—that is, shift the blame back to you, belittling and devaluing you for the sole purpose of getting you to doubt yourself and reconsider your decision. Do not fall for this attempt to manipulate you either.

No matter their reaction, don't let the masks deceive you. In the next chapter, I will explain what masks of manipulation to expect when you break up with a narc so that you are armed for this war, because they will be coming at you pretending to be all kinds of soldiers.

chapter 8

what to expect when you leave

"The only way to win with a toxic person is not to play."

—Iyanla Vanzant

I want to prepare you for what is to come when you finally decide to end the relationship. If you know what to expect, you will be guarded against all the narcissist's tactics that they will use to try to keep you from leaving them.

what to expect from the narcissist

Throughout your relationship with the narc, you have seen all their calculated sides. They have been in control, and you breaking up with them and meaning it for real this time is going to throw them off-balance, and they will panic. They will use every tool in their toolbox to get you back under their spell, under their control, just so they can decide when it's over and discard you. I call this the "masks" that they put on in their act. Based on my years of research and experience, these masks can range from acting innocent to outrageous, and all are intended to confuse you, instill doubt, and regain the upper hand. The following describes all the possible masks I know of.

After each mask description, I include a story from a survivor to show a real-life narc's reactions to breakups. Perhaps you can relate to some of these stories. While each story aligns most with a specific mask I'm describing, you'll notice that many of them feature several masks. This is common, as narcissists often switch between masks—sometimes within the span of a single minute—depending on what they think will manipulate or control the situation most effectively.

angry mask

When you attempt to break up with a narcissist, a common initial reaction from a narc is anger. This mask involves rage, yelling, cursing, and hurling hurtful insults at you. They lash out because they feel their control is being challenged and threatened, which is highly unsettling for the narcissist. Their anger can be so intense that it may escalate from verbal and emotional abuse to possible physical violence. Understandably, this can scare you and make you question whether leaving is worth it. But just know that the narc is highly aware that if they evoke enough fear in you, you may back down from your decision and remain under their control.

HOW TO RESPOND

The best way to respond to the angry mask is to remain calm. Keep your responses short and remain composed. I understand it will be hard to not react to their hurtful words, but do not engage in the argument. If you do, it will only escalate their anger because narcissists thrive on emotional reactions. They love to see the control they have over your emotions. Do not give that to the narc. Repeat your mantra sentence, as we discussed previously, as often as you have to. Say nothing else. And, of course, stand firm with your decision. If you give the narc any sense of doubt or hesitation about your decision, they will see an open opportunity to manipulate you into staying.

ANGRY MASK—VIOLENCE TWIST

If the narc has a history of physical abuse, you need to either not break up with them in person or have a special exit plan in place. Never break up with a violent narcissist in private. If there is violence involved, it is essential to have a friend or family member join you for the talk or wait for you somewhere they can see you, as I explained earlier. If you have experienced violence in your relationship, it is important to plan your breakup talk in a public space. If they get violent regardless of your precautions, please get law enforcement involved. This is not something you should handle on your own. Again, if you have kids, ensure they are not present at the time of the breakup; they should be entirely somewhere else, not just in another room.

Tyler's Story

"When I told her I was leaving, she completely lost it. She grabbed the nearest glass and smashed it against the wall, screaming, 'You're not going anywhere! You think you can just walk away from me, you piece of shit?' When I tried to walk past her, she shoved me so hard I stumbled back. Her nails dug into my arm as she spat, 'You're a worthless coward, and no one will ever want you! Go ahead! Run away like the pathetic loser you are!' No one has ever had the power to hurt me like she did."

blaming mask

Remember how your narcissistic partner struggles to take responsibility for anything that goes wrong within your relationship? This is not about to change when you break up. Be prepared to be blamed. The narc may accuse you of the most absurd things, like you didn't love them enough, you're too demanding, you didn't try hard enough to make the relationship work, or you are sabotaging the relationship. Expect to be blamed for anything and everything! This is their attempt to make you question whether it's your fault the relationship isn't working, leading you to rethink your decision and stay.

HOW TO RESPOND

When they begin to blame you, try to let those blameful insults fly past you and do not acknowledge them. If you were really so bad in the relationship, then why would the narc now fight to stay with you and not break up with you sooner? The point is, you were none of those things, and the narc is simply trying to make you doubt yourself and take the focus off of them.

Hannah's Story

"I ended the relationship again—I desperately hoped this time was the last time. I had broken up with him a half dozen times before, but his hoovering would always get the best of me because of our trauma bond. He continues to contact me and blames me for everything he's done at my farm and how I didn't do anything for him. It fluctuates daily, or hourly, between his blaming me, lambasting me about all the ways I've been a horrible person, and telling me how much he loves me and wants to make it work."

superiority mask

Expect for your vulnerabilities to be weaponized and used against you. With this mask the narc will attack your self-esteem by belittling and demeaning you. You may hear things like, "You think you can do better than me? Try it." Or "You're nothing without me, and you'll see that soon enough." Or "I'm the best thing that ever happened to you, and you're throwing it all away." They want to make you feel small, unworthy, and insecure, leading you to believe that leaving them would be a massive mistake.

HOW TO RESPOND

Do not take the bait. Do not believe them for one second. Stay calm and remind yourself of your own strength, worth, and accomplishments. The narc is not a reliable judge of character; their perception of everyone and everything is skewed. You can ask someone who truly unconditionally loves you, or ask yourself. Write down all the things you love about yourself and hate about them before you break up with the narc. After the breakup, read that list to remind yourself of your worth and their toxicity.

Paige's Story

"When I told her I was leaving, she leaned back in her chair, a smug smile creeping across her face. 'Finally. I've been stuck with this dead weight for years.' She didn't yell or lash out—she didn't need to. Her words cut sharper than any scream, dismissing me like I was nothing. As I walked out the door, she called after me with a laugh, 'Good luck finding someone who'll put up with you and your ugly kids.' She was the queen of making me feel worthless."

shame mask

The shame mask is another aggravated mask they put on if the anger and superiority masks don't work. You may hear things like, "What's your family going to think of you breaking up again? You're already old!" Or "Someone like you will never find someone stupid enough to settle down with you."

HOW TO RESPOND

Again, don't take the bait! These comments are strictly designed to belittle you, hoping to make you feel worthless and insecure enough to come back around and stay with them. They want you to give up hope that there is anyone better out there, that there is anything more you deserve. But remember, if you were all those things, then they should be happy that you're leaving them, but this is their attempt to get you to stay. This means you can't be bad after all!

Naomi's Story

"After my teenage daughter told me that he had been inappropriately flirting with her, I immediately felt disgusted and angry. I impulsively texted him that I wouldn't tolerate his bullshit behaviors anymore, and this was the final line he had crossed. I told him I will go to the authorities. His response was insane. He replied, 'Your daughter actually hates you and you don't even know it. She was actually flirting with me. At least she is still attractive. Look at you. Your best years are behind you. And trust me, no one's lining up for what you have to offer. You're just another sad, washed-up woman.' His response was genuinely absurd: He showed no concern about the police, as he was too busy insulting me. To give you context, I'm only thirty-seven years old and I am super fit, as I am a gym instructor. His insults truly make no sense."

victim mask

With the victim mask, the narcissist puts on a fantastic, desperate attempt to play the victim. Suddenly the narc is pleading with you to stay by saying they cannot live without you or that you are abandoning them when they need you the most. They suddenly no longer appear to be this strong, grown-up person they always say they are but rather appear like a little child who needs love and support. This is an extremely emotionally manipulative tactic to get you to feel empathetic and compassionate for them. They may even use past traumas, illnesses, or any personal hardships that would make you feel like a cruel person for leaving them, leading you to feel like you must stay and save them. But where were they when you needed their love and support? Where were they when you were sick? They most likely weren't there. Remember that. This victim mask is just a show, and you need to try your best to see right through it.

HOW TO RESPOND

You will feel your heart beating faster while they promise they will change. You will want to believe them. Your heart will be saying things like, "Finally they get it. Let's just give them one more chance. It looks like they finally see how much I care." Do not let them fool your heart. It is not a real promise; it is empty words. Equally, if they say hurtful things to you and your heart drops to your stomach, also know that these are empty words of deceit, attempting to get you back under their control. Your heart is wonderful, but it is naïve and can only get hurt in this scenario, so protect it as much as you can. Tell it that just for today, you are taking over.

Sarah's Story

"When I finally broke up with my narc, he said I was a horrible person for abandoning him because I knew he had an abandonment wound from childhood. The exact moment I was leaving, he got down on his knees and said, 'Let's have a kid and get married, you can even ask my mom about how I asked her to shop for an engagement ring for you.' He didn't want kids, and he didn't want to get married to me, but he'd use that as a dangling carrot. That same night he went out on a date (he had been speaking to other women), and after a week they were officially together. He introduced her to his family and friends within the next month, proceeding to say I was a nasty, crazy bitch who was mentally damaged."

begging mask

If their overused victim mask no longer has an effect on you, they will attempt to get you to stay with the begging mask. They will make (empty) promises of changing for the better and maybe even admit to their wrongdoings. They will cry and beg with desperation to give them one more chance. They will praise you and say how much you mean to them, that you are the love of their life, and that they will never find someone like you again. They want to make you believe that they really, truly love and care about you. Isn't it ironic how they used to torture you by saying you would never find someone like them again, and now they are begging you to stay, implying they'll never find someone like you? It makes no sense, like everything the narc does. It's all just a tactic to get control back. Keep that in mind.

HOW TO RESPOND

Your narcissistic partner's empty promises are probably all you have wanted to hear during times of abuse. So now when the narc is crying and begging you to stay, the temptation is surely strong to do so. The begging mask is one of many masks that are hard to say no to. In this mask they suddenly seem truly human again, like they have a beating heart. Let me reassure you, though, that if you fall for this mask, they will revert to their old behaviors.

Irem's Story

"He exploded in anger when I first told him I was leaving. But then, like a switch had flipped, he was on his knees, begging me to stay. He pulled out a giant diamond ring and proposed right there, promising me the world. 'I can't live without you,' he sobbed, tears streaming down his face. I rejected him again and again, but he just kept crying, for hours, like his life depended on it. For a moment, it almost worked. Almost."

suicide mask

The suicide mask is probably the most manipulative tactic a narcissist can use. If the angry and victim masks do not work, they will revert to this one because they know it will instill the biggest amount of fear and guilt in you. Please be prepared for this one. They will tell you that if you leave, they can't live anymore and that you are the only one keeping them alive. Suicide threats should always be taken seriously, but with a narcissist it is tricky. They are most often bluffing and only do this to get you to stay because they know it will work. They do this to create immense pressure and responsibility on you for their well-being. They rely on the fact that you care enough not to let them come to harm, which traps you in the relationship out of fear for their life.

HOW TO RESPOND

If you fear that their threat of suicide is real, there are steps you can take to ensure they get the help they need without getting back together with them. Even if you don't feel it's real, you can follow these steps anyway to protect your conscience.

1. Inform their family and close friends that they have threatened suicide and that they need support.

2. Contact a suicide prevention hotline for guidance if you need to.

3. Through steps 1 and 2 you transfer all the responsibility to someone who should be taking care of them, such as a family member or friend. Once you have called or texted them, they are informed, so you have done enough and can walk away, even if they continue the threats.

4. Your ex is no longer your responsibility. They are no longer your job.

I know this seems heartless, but it is the only way for you to save yourself, which has to be the only priority for you right now. You can *never* save someone who actually wants to kill themselves, because they will always find a way to do it. But in my many years of work experience as a psychotherapist, I have never seen or heard of a narcissist actually kill themselves. They will threaten you and then have a short rebound, where if they notice you don't react as they want you to, they will simply revert to another mask. If you don't react, they usually and very quickly will get very angry and blame you, almost like they completely have forgotten their suicide threats. Of course, I cannot guarantee that this will never happen—if, for example, the narc also has other personality disorders that will make them psychologically fragile—but a true narcissist with NPD would never kill themselves for you or anyone else.

Allie's Story

"When I finally told him it was over, he got very angry and blamed me for everything under the sun, whether it made sense or not. He wouldn't let me speak, tried to chase me, and attempted to steal my phone so I couldn't call anyone. He told me he'd take the kids and that I wouldn't have a home. In between bouts of anger, he played the pity card. Before walking out the door, he threatened to kill himself—right after threatening to kill me."

hoovering mask

After you have broken up with the narc, expect them to try everything to pull you back in. This is called hoovering. In this phase, just like in the love-bombing phase, the narc will charm you, give you presents, make promises to change, and shower you with affection. They will reflect on all the good times you two shared by sending you old, sweet messages or photos. The narc will, without a doubt, sweet-talk you again. This loving behavior is what you have been missing for such a long time that if they show you the love, care, and attention you wanted throughout the whole relationship, it is hard to say no to it. This is dangerous, as your plan was now to go cold turkey on your addiction to them, but they are offering you another hit right in front of you. You're still missing them like hell, wishing the "better version" of them will come back, so it is extremely tempting to give in. Hoovering gives you an (empty) promise of exactly that. Often this strategy will work, even several times in a row, until you realize it's still a show and nothing changes for the long term. Some victims go back to their narc after months or even years, leaving healthy relationships, all due to their hope of their former partner returning to how it was in the beginning. Their promise of change will make you feel that incredible spark again and reignite hope for a better version of them.

HOW TO RESPOND

Please do not let them fool you. All of it is NATO (no action, talk only). Think of me as a little angel on your shoulder telling you to hold back. They will not go through with this! As soon as they have you back in their pocket, the evil narc will come right back out. This is when you need to be extremely careful! Let this book be a reminder for you that the empty hoover promises are temporary and only a manipulative attempt to gain back their control over you so that they can be the one deciding when to dump you. Usually this phase only lasts a maximum of several weeks before their abuse returns, yet often it just lasts a couple of days. *All the hard work you've been through, all the rough times, the weeks of crying in bed, the months of flashbacks—all of that was for nothing if you cave now. Please don't.*

Alex's Story

"A week after he found out I'd been on my first date since him, the texts started. The first was a picture of us at the beach laughing and smiling, and he wrote, 'Remember us? No one made me as happy as you did.' I didn't respond, but it wasn't easy. I had very mixed feelings about him texting me. The next text was a photo of the day we moved into our apartment. He wrote, 'We were supposed to build a life together. Don't throw it away over some stranger.' At first I was wondering how he knew I went on a date, and then I got angry because that meant he was getting information about my private life. Then I got angry at myself for caring that he cared. He knew that by texting me those photos he could get to me. It worked. Every picture brought back memories. It completely messed me up for a few days, to the point I stopped responding to the guy I had gone on a date with. In the end, I decided to not respond to either one of them. I needed time to process. But after a few days of ignoring my ex, he got angry and wrote, 'Good luck with that loser—you really downgraded, didn't you?' It was clear I made the right decision to not respond."

stalking mask

If nothing else worked and you have stayed strong in your opposition to the narc, they might turn to the illegal mask—stalking. Since they can no longer control you officially, they have to act on their obsession to control you unofficially. They will stalk you by constantly contacting you, obsessively checking your social media and commenting or DM'ing you, contacting your friends and family, or worst of all, showing up at your home or workplace constantly. This is extremely intimidating and can actually worry and scare you. If they catch you off guard, they get a chance to involve you in another conversation, where often victims give in and talk to them.

HOW TO RESPOND

Please be careful here not to engage in any conversation no matter what they say to entangle you and lure you right back into a dynamic that will cause you harm and distress. If you need to, get the police involved with a restraining order. Unfortunately, chances are they will most likely not leave you alone for a while.

Aubrey's Story

"When I was finally able to have the strength to pull away, it took a lot of effort. It took a friend to recognize the toxicity and point it out to me. When I finally broke up with him, he was relentless. He sent me miles of texts. When those didn't work, he moved to emails, multiple times a day. When that still didn't work, he went to acquaintances to try to convince them to help him see me. Even after all that, he ended up sitting outside my apartment building. I ended up getting a restraining order and cutting my hair, changing my hair color, and getting fake glasses. I also moved into a house with my name not attached at all, due to concerns for my safety. In all his written communication, it always went back and forth from anger to false promises, sweet-talking, gaslighting, and blaming. He tried everything. If it weren't for my friend, I know I would have fallen for it and gone back."

social sabotage mask

Since you were the one who ended the relationship, their ego and pride are damaged. Hurting their ego is the worst thing you can do to a narcissist. They will not let that slide. At this point, they will want to protect their public image while destroying yours. They will spread lies about you to your friends, work colleagues, even family members in an attempt to turn them against you. Often this works, as they are so unbelievably charming, and they pretend to be hurt while doing so. Here they will also use their victim mask, of course. They will be out to destroy your reputation, take away any happiness you seek, and break down your support system while gaining credibility with their sob story. Their goal is to make your life a living hell. If they can't have you, no one can. If you're not happy with them, you better not be happy without them.

This post-breakup mask will feel like an all-out war. You desperately want to protect your image as the honest one, and I understand your urge. You must be smart here and override your longing with your mind. Remember, if you give them any opportunity for a power play, they will win. If you are desperate to look good in front of people, they will exploit that. It fuels their fire to start a dramatic war.

HOW TO RESPOND

You might be thinking, "All I want is to hold them accountable for their bullshit! I don't want them getting away with it *again*!" I get that! But be the wiser one here. Let them get away with it. Let them do their thing and "steal your friends" away. Anyone who chooses the narc over you was never really your friend, so thank them for showing you. And as far as you are concerned, people will remember how easily you let them go, how you didn't put up a fight over who has the better image, and how you walked away with grace while they tried tearing your name apart and dragging you through the mud. In the end, you will be the winner; you will be the one people respect (even if they do so silently). Channel your inner Buddha or Zen expert, and let your wise self take the lead!

Claim your power by practicing patience—do not react to *anything provoked by your ex*. When the narc tries to provoke you through some form of contact, wait. I suggest taking a three-day pause before responding to anything you hear from someone about them. *Never, ever reply to the narc directly.* If you are doubted by friends and family, let it go. Real loved ones will stand behind you during these difficult times.

The less you engage, the more frustrated the narc will become. Eventually your friends and family with recognize the narc as the one who creates drama while you do nothing to feed it, and the narc's energy source will run out. This will lead them to find a new target and move on from you more quickly. You are the survivor of abuse here, and you know it; you don't need to prove it to anyone else. *You're the only one who needs to believe yourself and you need to wholeheartedly work on that.* Nothing else. Everything else will fall into place.

Remember, friends who doubt you during your worst times are not real friends! Real friends should always lift you up, especially when you are doubting yourself or being attacked by a narc.

Shirin's Story

"He is still in shock that I left and is telling everyone he doesn't know who I am anymore—because I finally stood up for myself! He's told our five children that I abused him and was only after his money, even though I left with nothing. He's still living in the marital home while the kids and I are crammed into a two-bedroom apartment. It's cramped and incredibly stressful for the six of us. He knows where we live and has threatened to take the kids, calling me an unfit mother."

new supply mask

When all their other tactics have failed, they will try to hurt you by getting into a new relationship and flaunting it in front of you and others. This is meant to truly wound you, and they will succeed with it. They will post pictures showing how amazing their new supply is, and they will make sure to display public happiness anywhere they can. They will hit up your favorite bar and walk their dog in your dog park. This is their final attempt to make you feel jealous, question your worth, and regret your decision to leave. They want you to think that they have the pure, perfect happiness with someone else so you can go home and blame the failed relationship on yourself. This often works and will instill massive self-doubt; you will wonder what the new partner has that you don't.

HOW TO RESPOND

It's so important to go *no contact* and stop any form of information exchange you have with them—through them, socials, friends, or family. Your ex will want you to believe they are perfectly fine without you and that you were the *only* problem all along. This new "perfect" relationship is just their first phase of the abuse cycle, and not what it seems! They will not be happy, as no one can be happy with a narc. Remember that. This poor new target! The narc most likely used the same tactics they used on you with their current target, and you should only feel sorry for the next one.

Livia's Story

"*My narc ex, who had been cheating on me on and off for months, ended up getting together with someone else two days after we broke up. He brought that person with him to our mutual friend's house that weekend and acted as if nothing had changed, even though we had been together for six years and friends with this group for two years. I was the one who introduced him to all these people. Suddenly it was like I was plucked out and she was dropped in, and no one batted an eye. No one asked any questions or checked in to see if I was okay. It left me feeling completely abandoned and, even worse, replaced.*"

NO CLOSURE

One truth about a narcissistic abuse relationship is that you will never, ever get closure from them. They would rather die than give that peace of mind to you. All survivors long for closure with their abuser. You want nothing more than a happy ending where you can amicably part ways. Unfortunately there is no way to get closure from a narcissist. But you don't need them for it. "True closure comes from within," as Jackson MacKenzie states in his book Psychopath Free. *Once you realize that, you need to focus on cutting your emotional ties to your abuser and stop waiting for them to help you let go. They never will.*

Once you realize that your abuser is like acid for you—they will burn away everything they touch—it will be a bit easier to let go. It takes a long time (much longer than standard breakups), and it's not a linear journey, but it's worth it in the end.

Searching for closure will result in the narc having another opportunity to twist and turn the truth, destabilize you, and push you down even further than you already are. They will engage in the usual behaviors: not accepting any responsibility, blaming everything on you, engaging in circular conversations, or even trying to pull you back into their life just to drop you again. The bottom line: Trying to get closure from them cannot result in anything good for you. The only beneficiary of a closure talk is the abuser—and their ego—but never you.

I have made the Healing Your Heart series that you can find in the resources section at the back of this book. This includes a wonderful meditation that allows you to cut the energetic cord to your ex without ever having to see them. It really helped me and many of my clients in the past. This meditation was given to me by one of my favorite meditation experts and appreciated therapist colleague—one with an angelic voice and aura: Lily Olsen. It truly did its magic for me, and I would love to share it with you.

Chrisa's Story

"After a lot of counseling and putting things into perspective about why I was attracted to him, I managed to get over him. A few months ago, I tried to give closure by seeing him and explaining that there's no need to fight or anything. It was the worst idea ever. He ended up calling me horrible things. I was shocked, but at the same time relieved that I didn't feel the need to explain anything to him, like I had done for the past five years."

This list covers every mask that you can expect coming from the narc. Unfortunately, being prepared for their reactions is only half the struggle. You also need to prepare for your own reactions. I'm not sure which part is harder.

what to expect from yourself

The emotional reactions you might have to all their masks will be hard to deal with. The feelings that arise will most likely trick you into thinking that the pain and torture you go through while being with them is less than the pain you will feel when you leave them for good. You may face the impulsive urge to run back to them and mend things.

relapsing and taking them back

Statistically speaking, it can take up to seven times to successfully break up with a narcissist. I realize this number is depressing and not very encouraging, but this book aims to be part of the reason you will outshine the statistics.

Let's break down this statistic. Why seven times? Well, because the narc is sneaky like a fox in getting you to believe them and give them another chance. You now know that they have a collection of masks they will use on you, and chances are that one of them has worked or will work to their benefit. That doesn't mean that you are naive or stupid; you're human. It's natural to want to mend a rupture with your intimate partner. That is a healthy attribute empathetic people carry. When the narc *seems* to provide a peace offering, you will want to take it. Be very careful and attentive here. *If you manage to simply observe their behavior for their actions rather than empty promises, you will see that there is nothing there of substance.* They will never change for good, only temporarily, so they can further manipulate and control you. If you go back because you fell for their charm in their hoovering mask or felt sorry for them with their victim mask or any other mask fooled you—do not beat yourself up for it. Expect to have a *very* short period of time when the narc is super-nice and charming again. This will make you feel and experience several things. The anxiety will suddenly seem gone. You will be able to freely breathe again and find comfort as you calm down. You will feel the heavy cloud of darkness that was accompanying you suddenly lift. You will feel that color is back in your black-and-white world and things start to make sense again. Perhaps you can even concentrate on work, your kids, or any other part of your life that is not your partner. You will have your heart full of hope and positivity—feeling safe again like you haven't in a long time. You will find yourself smiling again. You might be thinking things to yourself like, "Clearly all these self-help books are bullshit, and no other source of guidance fully understands my relationship"; or "My relationship is special, my partner is different, and I might just be that one lucky person whom they love enough to change for"; or "Love can change people with narcissistic personality disorder."

Unfortunately, if we stick to statistics, all those thoughts are delusional and unrealistic. You are not special to them, and they will not change. Change of the villain is simply something we all want to see happen, as it's something that's been fed to us by fairy tales, Disney, and romantic movies. This is real life, and this is dealing with a personality disorder. *There is no happy ending to your story with them, only a happy ending to your story without them.*

Mark my words: This phase will not last more than several weeks, tops. Usually it only lasts a couples of days. Either way, I cannot stress this enough: *this reunited phase will not last.* Do not let these few days or few weeks of being back together without drama trick you into thinking the narc has changed and opening your heart again. Remember, you need to observe their actions, not solely believe their words, and test them for consistency.

In all my years as a therapist, in every narc-abuse couple I have accompanied, the narcs express countless promises to change. Their hoovering was unbelievably believable (even I almost believed them!), and they lured their partners back in plenty of times with fake promises—just to break their hearts and trust all over again. *I have not once met a couple where the narcissist changed for good.*

Relapsing doesn't mean you've failed. It's often part of the healing process. Sometimes you need to go back for another round and receive another metaphorical punch to the gut, slap to your face, or bash to your head to understand that this is not going to get you where you want to go.

After the very short colorful high, things will go black again. This realization is especially painful. It is so hard to bear the disappointment you feel in them and in your decision-making. You will not want to believe that it's really happening again, especially after things seemed to be going so well and felt so right. Instead of denying the reality, you need to keep your eyes open and look straight at it. Reassess your boundaries and remind yourself who you are and what you've been through. Remember your lists—take them out and read them. Any boundary you had in the past that they have eroded, put it back up. For example, if your partner restricted you from seeing your family and isolated you, then use this time to strictly enforce this boundary by planning time with your family without them, and watch how they react.

After building up your boundaries again, make sure this time around you're not doing it alone. It's so much harder when you're by yourself. Instead, surround yourself with people who truly care about you and can help you create an exit plan and stay grounded in the meantime. It's always good to get outside opinions, because people who love you will be much stricter with the narc than you will ever be. They will unravel the lies and deceit faster than you can.

At this point, if you're still mad at yourself for being back with them, drop it. Being angry and unforgiving with yourself only adds to your plate and doesn't serve you. The only way to grow is to forgive yourself for being back in this place. Forgiving means holding compassion in your heart for making a mistake, but it also means realizing that it was a mistake and making a promise to yourself to learn from it.

the chemical addiction of your trauma bond

It's not all willpower and being strong; there is also a chemical explanation to relapse that is often the reason people fail with their plan to leave their abuser.

Michael's Story

"I caught her in lies, stories that didn't make sense. My body felt electric and filled with anxiety. I know she wasn't treating me well, but I ignored it. I forgot about all the bad and focused on the good. We were on and off for almost three years. I was literally addicted to her. When we would break up, all I could think about was her and where I could've gone wrong. It had me going back every time."

Now that you broke up, as with any addiction, you're still craving your ex. Your brain tries to navigate the emotional low you are experiencing post-breakup while it longs for the highs you used to get from your ex in between. It takes time for your brain to recalibrate. To heal, you need to understand the specifics of the neurotransmitters created during the abuse. I will explain the five main neurotransmitters and hormones involved in a toxic relationship so you understand why it's so hard to break free from it.

The first hormone is the stress hormone, cortisol. In a toxic relationship, cortisol is constantly released due to continual conflict, manipulation, and emotional abuse. This creates a heightened state of stress that you can literally see in your bloodwork. Overproduction of cortisol leads to anxiety, a weakened immune system, insomnia, and weight gain. If you remain in this state for a while, your body begins to get used to this level of stress and eventually has a hard time living without it.

The second hormone that kicks in during stressful periods is adrenaline, also known as epinephrine. It's the hormone that is linked to our fight-or-flight response in moments of fear or intense anger. There are many moments in a relationship with a narc that will have you feeling this type of physical tension, and the temporary calmness that follows never lasts long. This hormone can become further addictive because it creates a sort of rush in your body, even if it is strenuous and harmful.

The third player in the chemical dependency rush is the feel-good neurotransmitter dopamine. Dopamine is released when you eat chocolate, have great sex, play sports, or anything else that is linked to the brain's reward-and-pleasure system.

Narcissistic relationships are awful, but not all bad, and the good moments can be so wonderful that you are grateful for their attention and affection. Those short-lived happy moments release dopamine, but the rewards are unpredictable. In the beginning phase of love-bombing, dopamine spikes extremely high, so once your narc drops you to the devaluation phase, you are busy trying to recreate the positive and get that boost of dopamine again. This loop keeps you chasing that ever-so-desired sense of happiness, despite the overall sense of sadness.

Oxytocin is the fourth important hormone in this cocktail. It's the bonding hormone mothers get when they breastfeed or lovers get when they experience true intimacy. Your body releases oxytocin with every positive interaction with your narcissist, further encouraging feelings of attachment, even if they are short-lived.

Serotonin is the last ingredient in the chemical bond. It regulates moods and emotions. When circumstances are uncertain, like they are with a narc, the fluctuations in serotonin levels often lead to anxiety or even depression. The constant up and down creates a chemical imbalance, making you crave the narcissist more, despite their harmful nature.

You will experience most of these hormones in a healthy relationship, as you can have fights and moments when adrenaline or cortisol rises; and you can have great moments of intimacy, which spike your oxytocin, serotonin, and dopamine. The key difference is the intensity of the hormone response, the empty handouts of oxytocin (because they make you trust the narc, but then the narc abuses that trust), and the unreliable releases of these hormones. You are merely focused on keeping up, rather than feeling calm and enjoying it, as you would with a typical relationship. Due to the sheer intensity and unpredictability, your brain becomes trauma bonded and chemically dependent on the narcissist. *There is no drug stronger than another human being.*

Unlike a healthy relationship where things are just no longer working out—*the narc* is the true source of your pain. The narcissist is causing you all this anguish. So going back to the creator of your pain is simply not the answer in any scenario. You have to get as far away from that source of pain as soon as possible. Let me share the feelings that are most likely to hit you so that you can be prepared as best you can. Two things to remember here:

1. Knowing that your emotional reactions are predictable validates that you are normal, *not* crazy.

2. Anticipating the emotional reactions that might hit you decreases their power over you.

grief, sadness, and depression

There is a depth to grief and sadness after an abusive relationship that goes unmatched. The extreme contrast between your fantasy and the harsh reality makes the grief so much sharper. Despite the toxicity and suffering in the relationship, you are still sad about losing the "what could have been." You have probably never been so deeply invested in any other relationship as the one with a narc. The loss of your potential perfect partner can kick-start a major depressive episode. You might not want to get out of bed in the morning, you're unmotivated for hygiene, you stop eating or overeat, you stop sleeping or sleep all day. You lose a sense of yourself and don't recognize who you are anymore. The pain may overshadow everything for some time. But this feeling of devastation is showing you the way. It is a sign—your sign—that you don't deserve their abuse. You are grieving the dream of an idealized relationship you once believed in; you're not actually grieving them. You didn't actually lose anyone real because the person you fell for didn't exist.

WHAT TO DO

It is super important to seek professional help! Therapy will tremendously increase your chances of healing. It is extremely important to reach out to someone who is experienced in intimate partner abuse and narcissistic personality disorder. Without the necessary experience, they can actually do more harm by giving you a false diagnosis and treating you inappropriately (e.g., diagnosing borderline personality disorder when actually you have C-PTSD). If you are not sure, ask them and check their references online. All therapists should have a list of their areas of expertise on their website. If you can't seem to make it out of your house or get out of your pajamas, then start with an online therapist and do your sessions from home. I offer online therapy and group sessions worldwide if this book resonates with you.

The end goal to overcoming the deep depression that follows a breakup with a narcissist is breaking free from the victim mindset. This does not happen automatically. You need to put in the work. When you do, it will happen naturally over time. When you are ready, you will realize that you are no longer a victim. Just like the caterpillar turning into a butterfly, what you have become is a survivor. Keep telling yourself this: "I am a survivor!" *Victims aren't able to act; survivors are.* The question now becomes how you will use this awful experience to reclaim your life.

Some things that may help are journaling, meditation, exercise, daily positive affirmations, eating healthy meals, and staying hydrated. There are also effective medications that can help you overcome an acute crisis in your life. Antidepressants or antianxiety medication can be a lifesaver in times like these. However, antidepressants can only take away your depressive *symptoms*; you still must put in the work to heal from your trauma. Medication simply gives you the strength you need to actively work on the problem yourself.

If nothing is helping and you are contemplating suicide, *put this book down immediately and seek professional help.* Call a trusted friend or family member and tell them how bad you are feeling. Call a suicide hotline or an ambulance or go to a hospital emergency department for immediate support.

CHECK-IN

When you are in such a deep sad place, your inner voice will tell you that the narc is the only person that you need right now. It will tell you that they will fix how you are feeling. And they would—for a couple of days, before they hurt you again. Don't forget, they are the source of your current pain. Your mind is playing tricks on you. You need to seek your long-term goal (an abuse-free life!) instead of short-term gratification (giving in to your longing for them). You cannot heal in the same place where you were hurt!

emotional exhaustion

An intimate relationship with a narcissist leaves you emotionally, physically, and mentally drained. Every moment spent worrying, anticipating their next outburst, fighting for their love and attention, or endlessly trying to please them has robbed you of your energy. Once you actually pulled through breaking up with them, often this exhaustion hits you even harder. It's like the feeling you get when you have been extremely stressed for a long period of time, where you had to push through for a high-intensity period before you went on a vacation. Often, during this long-awaited vacation, you get sick because now you no longer have to function. Similarly, now you are able to relax after having to endure all the abuse with your body's last strength. I am not saying that you feel it's relaxing when you break up with a narc, but your body does. By not having them around you, your body is allowed to stop producing all your stress hormones. Since you are no longer walking on eggshells, your cortisol levels drop, and this helps your physical body calm down and relax. It's quite common to get the flu, strep throat, gastritis, or other common infections at this point because your immune defenses go down.

You might possibly even find yourself sleeping much more than before. You would intuitively think that after the stressor leaves your life, you will feel free and at ease. Unfortunately, not having to worry and preempt the narcissist's behavior doesn't always feel good. Isn't this ironic? It can actually feel extremely unsettling and strange, because you are so used to constantly being on edge. Once the storm leaves your life and you are left feeling a sense of calm, you feel a big void. It can actually feel scary and threatening to not have anything to do. You may feel unworthy. This sounds so paradoxical, but it is what C-PTSD/NVS does to you. So, if suddenly you feel you have no purpose in your life, understand that this feeling is common. Common, yes, but not true. You have a higher purpose than chasing a narcissist's mood around. Adding to the unfamiliar, unsettling void, you might experience intrusive thoughts like, "Why did I allow this abuse in my life for so long?" These thoughts are extremely critical and painful, further adding to your exhaustion.

WHAT TO DO

When emotional exhaustion happens, it is important not to resist, and allow yourself this time to *not* function. Your body is allowed to take a break. Just try to take care of yourself as best you can with proper rest, nutrition, exercise, and hydration. Try calming activities such as yoga or craft projects.

On the bright side, the exhaustion will not last if you let it be there for now and accept it. If you can, take a bit of time off to let your physical body settle. Not too long, as you will recover much quicker if you are working or have something different to do during the day than thinking about your ex. Also, chronic psychosomatic pains and symptoms you may have experienced during the abuse will slowly or abruptly stop. This is a sign from your body that you are beginning to recover and a beautiful step in the right direction. Embrace it and see it as another milestone.

shame, guilt, and confusion

A common reaction to a breakup with a narcissist is feeling shame and guilt—shame for staying even though you were enduring abuse, and guilt for still loving them or even wanting them back. Sometimes you might even experience feeling sorry for *them*. They are fabulous fakers who made you believe so strongly that some of these things are real. You might also have the urge to be there for them. These feelings are common and show that everything *you* felt was real. *Still, you cannot let these feelings be your guide in this dark time.* Allow yourself to feel these emotions but know that you cannot act on them. Going back is not the answer.

During this confusing emotional chaos, it is very important to hold compassion for yourself by allowing the emotions to go through you. When you disregard a feeling or label it negatively (e.g., "I am so stupid for feeling shame!"), you are not acting with compassion. If a child told you they feel so stupid because they messed up their homework, you wouldn't bash them. You would uplift them by saying something like, "It's okay to feel disappointed, but you did your best! It's in the past. Just try to do better next time." That is the same attitude you need to hold for yourself. Be the adult that the little one inside you now needs! Instead of criticizing yourself further, hold a compassionate attitude (like toward that child) for yourself. Try to hug yourself tight for at least thirty seconds at least once a day, and say something sweet to yourself, such as "This is a very tough time. It's okay to feel like this. This too will pass, and I will get through it!" Understand that you need to be your own nurturing parent/best friend right now. Be patient as you wait for these difficult feelings to pass.

Also, it is completely natural to miss a partner after a breakup—it is all part of the process of breaking up with someone you cared about. I understand that missing your abuser can feel wrong, especially because they've deeply hurt you. You might think, "Why would I miss someone who caused me so much pain?" But this feeling stems from the trauma bond you have with the narc.

Feeling like you miss them is not a sign for you to take them back but a sign to show you the massive power the manipulations still hold over you.

Often you will think to yourself that you never, ever want them back, but you *still* miss them. This contradiction will surely cause shame and confusion. You need to look at what you are *actually* missing. You are most likely missing the person you wanted them to be or the person they were pretending to be in the beginning. You are missing the potential that you believed in, the idea of them, the thought of their role in your life—everything you projected onto them. That person never actually existed. You can say to yourself, "I miss my version of them. That's okay, but I do not want them back!" Keep repeating this like a mantra. Breaking a trauma bond requires therapy and time. It isn't something that will disappear in a week. You have to put in the work and really want to get past it.

WHAT TO DO

Redirect these feelings of shame and guilt by reminding yourself of the abuse and allowing yourself to get angry. You were manipulated and controlled. This is *not* your fault. Turn these feelings of shame and guilt (which is anger at yourself) into anger at the abuser (explained on page 166). Allow yourself to be furious, but don't act on it.

INNER-CHILD EXERCISE

I would like to introduce a short inner-child exercise that I love to do in times like these to help release these negative feelings. Go back in time to a scene you remember when your younger self was experiencing the feelings you are feeling right now. Choose a scene where you were very hurt and feeling shame, sadness, or guilt for what happened. You might be feeling guilty for accidentally or purposefully hurting someone or for breaking something valuable. You might feel shame for acting out in a "bad" way. You might feel upset that things didn't go the way you wanted them to and nobody cared about it. All of those are okay. Just find a scene that comes to mind.

Now, connect with your younger self by closing your eyes and imagining your younger self feeling the feelings you are encountering right now. Look at your little one and see the scene around them. Imagine all that's there, and see it in front of your eyes. Where are you? Who is with you? What are you feeling exactly? Are you crying? What is happening in that scene? Once you've got all that, step into that scene as your adult self now and comfort and console your little one until they are no longer crying, angry, sad, or experiencing discomfort. Hug them, talk to them, cuddle them, play with them, and explain things to them that are relevant. Have that conversation and be sweet to them, giving them exactly what they need but didn't get from anyone else back then. Once they are smiling and feeling light again, you can send them off to play and tell them that they are not alone anymore, that from now on you are here to protect them. Once you feel good walking away, release that scene and go about your day. You will notice a small amount of peace flow through you every time you do this exercise. The more you practice, the better it will help you feel.

anger and rage

The most natural emotion that comes after going through shame and guilt is anger. It's what I would prefer you to feel. *Anger is your biggest friend when going through a toxic breakup.* This anger will save you from yourself. When you're reflecting on your relationship (purposely or with intrusive thoughts), you will replay scenes of abuse, manipulation, and betrayal. All these memories will trigger all sorts of emotions, but if you're lucky, they will trigger anger. Why lucky? If you are still in the shame-and-guilt phase, you are doubting and hating yourself, but if you are in the anger phase, you are directing your emotions toward the right target: the narcissist, not yourself. When you're angry, you cannot simultaneously be sad. Of course, all these emotions come intertwined, and often chaotically so. But again, whenever you're mad and angry—be grateful. Don't try to be a "good person" by minimizing your anger. Instead, make sure you allow yourself to really *feel* that rage against this horrible human who has put you through so much. Use it to close all your chapters with them. Leave them behind.

WHAT TO DO

If you get yourself truly worked up, possibly even developing physical symptoms, try doing something physical to release them, like kickboxing, running, or hitting a pillow and screaming at it with death metal playing in the background. Whatever you do, let it out (in a nonharmful way!). Do not seek revenge on your ex! You can fantasize about it: Write your revenge plan in a diary, record a mad song, draw a killer cartoon, or even hurt a *Sims* character that you created to look like your ex. All of that is allowed, but remember: Your ex is absolutely irrelevant! *Your ex is now your past.* This is the present and your future. These are your emotions now. Own them, be creative with them, and let them flow through you. Just like any other emotion, anger will also pass. But make sure your anger is directed at the right target, and not at other people around you. It is perfectly natural to experience rage when people do not believe the depth of your story, so make sure you only tell people who will be supportive. If they disappoint you with their reaction, move on to someone who will show up for you and who believes you.

erosion of identity (self-doubt)

After going through emotional abuse for a long time, you may no longer trust anything or anyone, even yourself. You may wonder whether you can trust your gut feelings, which you overrode for a long time in order to function in the relationship. This part of abuse is called identity erosion, and it happens when your narc systemically undermines your confidence, self-worth, and autonomy with their manipulations and abuse tactics. They take these away by gradually weakening your sense of self throughout the relationship. You are left doubting your values, beliefs, and identity. This causes huge trust issues. You have lost not only yourself but also your ability to believe in yourself. You might feel a deep sense of despair, missing the person you once were and fearing you can never be them again—but you can.

WHAT TO DO

The most important task now is taking control of your narrative. Don't tell yourself the sob story; tell yourself the truth: You were manipulated by a con artist and now you need to rebuild. With the help of a journal, start redefining who you are. Focus on your strengths, dreams, and goals. Reconnect with yourself by spending time doing what you love—things that matter to you separate from external influences—and revisiting old (or new) hobbies and relationships with friends and family that serve your goal. Establish boundaries with yourself, and don't let people into your life who do not serve you in a positive way. Whenever you doubt yourself or make a "wrong" decision, practice self-compassion by connecting with the little one who needs your comfort. Healing from identity erosion is considered a lifelong process, but with the self-awareness you now have, you can build a stronger version of yourself than you ever were before. Don't forget that autonomy is key! Whenever you can, be autonomous. Make your own decisions, and do not think about what others will think.

A classic narrative that often creeps into a survivor's mind is "They never loved me; it was never real." This statement will do nothing for you except make you feel bad. Change the narrative (and soothe your memory). They loved you—deficient as they are—as best they could. That deficient love is not enough. Ruminating about whether their love was real is pointless. You deserve sufficient love from someone whole.

trust issues and anxiety

Through identity erosion comes trust issues—not only with yourself but also with family and friends as well as any new relationships. It feels like you can never trust anyone again—and you don't want to try. You're upset and embarrassed that this happened to you, that you have lost yourself in the process, and that you gave yourself up for a completely lost cause. All of that makes sense and is natural to feel! The end of a toxic relationship can leave you feeling uncertain and unsafe with anyone, including yourself. The mere fact of trusting someone again feels scary.

Anxiety will manifest itself in this period of time, as you are still on edge, waiting for the next bad thing to happen. Usually in this phase, the threat is real because narcissists do not like to give up easily and will often hoover you, stalk you, or even threaten you. Yet often you will feel anxious even when there is no real threat present and the narcissist has started leaving you alone. You will remain hypervigilant post-breakup; it will take a while to wean away. The sense of not knowing what volatile and inconsistent behavior or outburst will come from your ex leaves a lasting imprint on your nervous system, even after the relationship has ended. It's like your body stays stuck in that hyperalertness, making it impossible to trust new experiences. This broken sense of security is a perfect place for more anxiety to creep in. Since your self-doubt is so deeply instilled, you worry about missing warning signs in the future. You are locked in protective mode trying to shield yourself from any potential harm. Healing as always is a gradual process, and you need to be patient with yourself so you can rebuild your trust in your instincts. Both anxiety and trust issues will not vanish overnight, but they can soften up if you are good to yourself.

WHAT TO DO

The most important part of working through trust issues is to talk about it. Talk about it as much as you need to in order to work your way through it, especially in a private or group therapy setting. Writing it down really helps. Online forums can help. Don't forget that many people are in abusive relationships and may truly feel inspired by your story! Your story could be the reason they actually leave their abuser. Anything you can do to get it out helps. Explain your story to your loved ones, but make sure you maintain boundaries where you need them to be right now. Be in control of when and to whom you tell your story. Try not to do this late at night in order to give your mind time to settle down before you go to bed.

fear of the unknown

Starting over without the narcissist might feel daunting. You are now facing the unknown. That can feel like running into a pitch-black forest, not knowing what to expect. It may even feel like you're in a horror movie, where you never know what is about to jump out and scare you. This is understandable but not necessarily true. Chances are high that the unknown is better than your life of abuse. The unknown may be a beautiful, heartwarming place where you find a new job, a new city, a wonderful new partner, and have an amazing life!

Still, it is common to have fearful thoughts about being alone: "What if I can't find anyone else and I will be alone forever?" "How can I start over? Nobody will want me." Do not fear being alone because of the lies your narc has fed you. The narcissist has made you feel like no one else will care for or love you like they do and, in a twisted way, they are right. Thank God. Here's why: Healthy partners will not engage in the same manipulative, fake-but-magical way a narcissist does. A healthy partner will truly care for you and love you authentically by offering genuine affection and respect without a hidden agenda of manipulation and control. The realness of authentic affection might not seem as exciting and contagious as a narc's love-bombing at first. This is the reason behind people falling for narcissists. The quick thrill ride is just so tempting. When you are making the next decision for your love life, choose feeling calm and safe rather than immediately excited.

WHAT TO DO

Choose optimism, not pessimism. Choose to see the glass half-full. You now have every opportunity everyone else has too. It is your opportunity to take control of your life and guide it toward your happy place. It may not feel like it right now, but being alone is a blessing in disguise. When we are alone, we have nothing left to focus on except ourselves. This is the perfect opportunity for serious self-growth, as you are now the one in control of your life. It offers an immense opportunity to learn about yourself, grow personally and spiritually, and make meaningful changes for the better.

If you are financially dependent on your ex, or if they scammed you out of money, you might be overwhelmed with thoughts of having to budget, find employment, apply for unemployment, or ask for help from others. Being in this difficult place is scary, but it will not last if you start working at it. Learning how to financially support yourself (and your children) is achievable and a powerful step toward freedom from your ex. Don't allow this fear to paralyze you (victim mode); instead, use it to give you the necessary energy to fight against it (survivor mode). Seek out resources to help you gain (or regain) your financial independence.

relief, hope, and empowerment

Not everything after a breakup is negative. In fact, being free from the toxic influence and control of a narcissistic partner will bring the color back into your life. This is where true transformation begins. The light in your eyes that your narcissist had dimmed will shimmer again. Suddenly, when you don't expect it, you'll feel a glimpse of hope that you can recover, and *you will*. You'll grow stronger, more resilient, and empowered enough to rebuild your life. The freedom from the narc is an amazing opportunity to find yourself again, rediscover who you were and who are you now, and thrive. Once you get through all the painful ups and downs of the breakup, you will find yourself feeling a sense of relief as well as hope and empowerment.

WHAT TO DO

Use your newfound sense of hope and empowerment as a source of strength. Instead of letting the pain of the breakup consume you, channel that pain into something great. Take your pain and turn it into power. Let it fuel your transformation! I love to quote Manifestelle, who always says, "Don't get mad, get paid." I believe in turning breakup pain into something creative, something that can feel extremely empowering. If you are a writer, write a book. If you're a dancer, choreograph something awesome and put it on TikTok. If you love to paint, sell some art online. If you're a poet, go to the next poetry slam. If you don't want to focus on money, use this quote metaphorically. "Don't get mad, get paid" just means using the energy of something bad and transforming it into something good. You could help out at an animal shelter, give out food to the homeless, or volunteer at a hospital. The point is to steer your energy toward something that makes the world a better place. Imagine yourself thriving after your breakup, doing some good with the energy of your pain instead of letting it define you.

Breaking up with a narcissist can feel like the death of a loved one. If you allow yourself to feel what this person has done to you, it is not possible to keep them in your life; your healthy self-esteem won't allow it. It is essentially the death of your rose-colored-glasses' version of your narcissist. Drawing on well-known grief models, I've developed a narc-breakup recovery model, the subject of the next chapter, to show you the specific stages of your pain in order to hold your hand when times get rough. All these emotions are very typical, and you are not alone with them.

chapter 9

recovery after your breakup

"Rock bottom became the solid foundation on which I rebuilt my life."

—J. K. Rowling

The original model of grief after losing a loved one was first described by Elisabeth Kübler-Ross in 1969 in her book *On Death and Dying*. In 2016, Shannon Thomas revised Kübler-Ross's model in her book *Healing from Hidden Abuse: A Journey through the Stages of Recovery of Psychological Abuse* to address grief stages after abusive relationships. I further tweaked their research and applied it specifically to narcissistic relationship breakups with my Kastner's 5R model of recovery after narcissistic abuse.

Kastner's five Rs of recovery after narcissistic abuse

After years of research and more than a decade's work with survivors of narcissistic relationships, I have developed my own recovery model specific to narcissistic breakups. I call it "the 5 Rs of recovery":

1. Rupture 2. Release 3. Rebuild 4. Rise 5. Radiance

My phases are designed to help you navigate the chaos of healing from a toxic breakup with a narcissist specifically. You are most likely going to be emotionally thrown back and forth between these phases, and that is perfectly natural. Healing from a toxic relationship takes more out of you than a regular breakup. Use this knowledge about the phases of this kind of breakup to your advantage and add it to your toolbox of wisdom. This will allow you to have a smoother transition into healing.

Remember, once you've run away from your rotten narc, you will experience these 5 Rs of recovery before reaching lasting resilience. Let's look closely at each phase.

1. rupture

During this phase, you are feeling completely torn, like a rupture has been made to so many aspects of your life. It feels like there is a rupture inside of you—the war between your heart longing for your ex versus your head telling you to leave this toxicity. There is a rupture in your relationship—they are not the person you thought they were. There is a rupture in your future vision—you can no longer build your original vision with your ex; you have to create a new one. Last but not least, there is a rupture in your self-image—you have most likely lost parts of your identity and often doubt yourself.

A breakup with a narc will leave a significant tear in all important aspects of your life. These tears cause intense pain and deep disappointment in life while creating a massive void within you. Splitting away from yourself, your partner, your past, and your future plans can leave you disoriented and raw, struggling to process reality. The pain is followed by emptiness, which allows extreme loneliness to creep in and tear you down further. This is often considered the hardest phase of recovery, but it also marks the start of something new: your self-discovery journey.

The following are the top rupture resolutions I suggest to my clients.

NO CONTACT
This is probably the absolute hardest step to take, but it is nonnegotiable. If you don't do this, you're set up for failure. If you only do this every now and then, you're set up for failure. Every form of contact will throw you right back to square one and

continue your suffering. There is nothing you can do to dismantle the importance of this step. Cutting off all forms of communication is essential to begin healing and breaking the emotional and psychological bond with your toxic ex.

Cynthia's Story

"I made the hardest decision of my life when I took that ring off, left it on the kitchen counter alongside the multitude of documents that revealed his lies, and packed my things before he returned from his trip. When he called, his words stung like salt in an open wound. He called me a coward, accused me of being crazy. 'Everything has an explanation,' he said, 'and you chose to run instead of waiting to hear me out.' But I knew better. If I had stayed, the lies would have shifted, his words would have twisted into gaslighting, and I would have been buried deeper under his deceit. The messages he sent afterward revealed everything: his blame-shifting, his half admissions, his acknowledgment that he shouldn't have lied or should have 'come clean sooner.' He also understood the power I held now, the proof I carried, and the threat it posed to his life of illusion. So, he kept his distance, choosing silence over confrontation."

If you find yourself struggling with following through with the no-contact rule, you are not alone. Statically speaking, a person will go back to their narc partner seven times, so don't beat yourself up for it. Just understand that without adhering to this rule 100 percent, you will not give yourself a chance to truly begin your healing.

Contact includes but is not limited to:

- Physical meetings in person (at each other's home or workplace, or waiting in places where the other one could go to, such as favorite bars, restaurants, etc.)
- Calls
- Voice messages
- Texts, WhatsApp, Snap, Signal, Viber, Telegram, Venmo, and other apps
- Email

- Letters
- Social media
- Talking to each other's (common) friends and family
- Talking to each other through family or friends acting as mediators
- Sending each other gifts
- Shared playlists on Spotify/Apple Music/YouTube

If you own any joint pets (say, you adopted the pet together and didn't already own it before the relationship), and the narc won't let you have that pet for good, unfortunately you have to take this bullet and let that pet go. I love my pets more than anything, but no pet in the world is worth continuing to choose an abusive relationship. You must put yourself first. If you think the narc will not treat your pet right, call animal services and see whether you can get adoption rights.

Kristin's Story, *Two Years Post-Breakup, after Not Cutting Contact*

"Even though we haven't spoken in months, it's like he's still pulling the strings. He knows exactly how to mess with me without even being there. He'll post some random, cryptic quote on Instagram, and suddenly I'm spiraling, wondering whether it's about me. Or he'll 'accidentally' send me a blank text, as if to remind me he's still lurking. The most ridiculous part? He sent me a playlist last week—an actual playlist—called 'Songs That Remind Me of Us.' Who does that? It's like he's out there crafting these tiny bombs to drop into my life just to see whether I'll explode. And the worst part is, I do. Every. Single. Time. He's nowhere near me, but he still finds these absurd little ways to make sure I'm never really free."

There is only one exception to the no-contact rule: If you share children with the narcissist, then you have to do what I call "limited contact"—limited to only the absolute essentials. Essentials are organizing the children and anything important (medical updates, school trips, practices, and so on) in the form of nonemotional texts. As soon as your ex tries to get you involved in a personal or emotional exchange, do not engage. The narc will beautifully put on one of their many masks and enjoy any reaction (whether positively or negatively charged) they can get out of you, because they want to control you. By provoking a reaction and getting one, they win. They will feel a rush of power while you will feel defeat. Don't let that happen. Still follow all the steps you can of the no-contact rule, just stick to one medium (e.g., text messages) and keep control over the depth of the exchange.

PARENTING WITH A NARCISSIST

If you have been trying really hard and your narcissistic co-parent never respects your boundaries (surprise!), you can get legal help from a lawyer or family court. Professional help through counselors or therapists who are experienced in narcissistic abuse can really help you work through all the rage and upset your ex will provoke in you. You are human, and it is understandable to want to react and sometimes fail to ignore them. You might feel that staying neutral will come across like you have no voice, but really it just demonstrates your power and self-discipline in holding back with them. That doesn't mean you should swallow your feelings, because you still need to let them out—just not with your ex! Rage rooms, rock concerts, or any high-adrenaline sports can help.

MINI SELF-CARE

I know at this point in time you are most likely not feeling able to properly take care of yourself, and you might spend 24/7 in your bed wasting away with your pain. That is understandable, but let me suggest something small that could help you step out of the rupture void and feel proud of yourself. Remind yourself that you are the only one responsible for yourself and that you can do your body a mini favor, even by taking the smallest steps toward healing. Eat something healthy, even if you don't feel like it. Don't starve your poor body; it has done so much for you, and you are still here! Sometimes you can add a fresh start to your day by simply taking a shower or washing your hair, which can make you feel like a different person. Taking a warm bubble bath at night to get out of the pajamas you've been wearing for days can settle your nervous system and ensure better sleep. Talking to one specifically chosen person to let them know how you're feeling also helps: It gives you the chance to voice your pain, and it gives them the opportunity to spend time uplifting you a bit! Don't further isolate yourself. Let loved ones know you need them to show up for you now, even if it's watching a movie and eating popcorn silently next to one another. You don't have to talk about your breakup or your ex. Whatever works to not feel so alone. Another small thing that makes a big difference is changing your bedsheets. I love how that can be a proud moment of freshness. All these mini self-care interventions will give you a small sense of renewal, a bit of comfort, and a bit of hope.

THERAPY

The first type of therapy I recommend is light therapy via a light lamp. You can order them online, and they can make a huge difference! Just ten minutes a day is proven to uplift your energy and spirit levels. The second type of therapy I recommend is talk therapy. If you're experiencing narcissistic victim syndrome or C-PTSD, the sooner you seek help, the better. Don't forget that you might not know you're suffering from one of these conditions, but a narc specialist could diagnose you properly and help accordingly. These conditions can worsen your current feelings of devastation, sense of loneliness, and loss of identity. So, it's very critical that you seek intervention now to prevent yourself from falling deeper into the rupture phase. If you're struggling to leave your home, remember that many therapists offer online sessions. No excuses! Don't let staying in bed stop you from getting the support you need!

Some people will experience the rupture phase fully, while others may feel numb. If you feel numb, that's okay. It's your body's way of protecting you by temporarily shutting down your emotions so you can function day to day. While this can be helpful, I still recommend seeking professional help. A therapist can provide a safe space for you to process your emotions and guide you toward the release phase.

2. release

During the release phase, you are able to release the emotional burden that you have been carrying around for so long. After the rupture phase, you now feel your suppressed emotions start to rise. Anything you didn't allow yourself to feel, or feelings you have been holding back such as anger at your narcissistic ex, might now pour out of you. This is the time and place to confront your pain head-on and no longer hold back tears, screams, or heartache. This phase is allowed to feel messy and raw. It is the right time to release that breath you have been holding for way too long, exhaling all the hurt, resentment, and frustration that has built up during that time.

Release is an emotional phenomenon, but as we know, body and mind are connected, so you might feel lighter as you purge the emotions that have been pent up. Doing so might feel like relieving yourself of a heavy weight, a sort of cleansing. That can feel liberating or scary, and both are okay! Let yourself take up some space to feel fully and know there is no right way to handle this phase. As long as you can feel the grip of your toxic ex releasing, you are going in the right direction. Honor your feelings as if they were your friends, not your enemies, because even when they overwhelm you, they are the most essential part of your healing journey.

The following are the top release resolutions I suggest to my clients.

PAIN HOUR

The pain hour is the practice of setting aside one hour every day, in a safe place where no one can disturb you so that you can feel your pain thoroughly and consciously. Get a journal and a pen, some arts and crafts—colorful pencils or other creative tools you love—an instrument if you play one, candles, pillows, blankets, tissues, your favorite playlist and a speaker, and anything else you might need. Now light your candles, prep your things, turn on your favorite music that matches your pain (sad/angry/hopeful) or an audio of your favorite poem and let it play. Set your alarm for exactly one hour. Then sit there and allow the pain to visit you. Welcome it in. Let it be there with you. For that whole hour, allow yourself to cry furiously, scream your lungs out, draw, play, write, or sing your thoughts, releasing the pain. Allow the universe to channel the pain through you and feel all of it. The more intense, the better. Once that alarm goes off, stop and move on with your day. Repeat as often as you need (maximum one hour a day) and for as long as you need. You can do any amount of time between fifteen minutes to an hour, whatever feels comfortable to you.

The point of this exercise is to give yourself an adult time-out to be your inner child with no guilt. Allowing yourself to feel your annihilating pain will soften its power over you. *You* decide the hour of when you invite it in, *you* decide what you do with it. The rest of the day, when you feel overwhelming pain or anger, tell yourself to contain yourself and tell your pain to pause for now and come back in your pain hour.

The perspective I want you to hold here is you taking back control over your life by controlling your emotions to a degree, without denying them. You take back autonomy and power over your life. You can be a true victim that hour and feel truly sorry for yourself when it is convenient. It is important to let yourself be a victim until you're tired of being a victim. Your time will come! Then, throughout the rest of the day, you can function (go to work, care for your children, and so on). It serves to let you continue life while not denying your pain but by accepting and welcoming it (during your pain hour). Get creative with it! Scream your favorite songs, cry, share it with a good friend who is going through the same thing—everything is allowed.

DETOX

Full detox is basically an important add-on to your no-contact strategy. Detoxing from your ex by going no contact helps but doesn't do the full trick. There are several little things you need to consider.

First I'd like to introduce the concept of the "analog" detox. An analog detox is physically removing anything and everything that reminds you of your ex. You do this by cleansing your space (bedroom, living room, and so on) of your ex. This includes removing pictures, reminders, letters, magnets, gifts, clothes, bedsheets—simply anything that belonged to your ex or reminds you of your time together needs to be removed. The point is to collect it all and remove it so that it is out sight and out of mind. If you don't have the strength to destroy it or throw it away, put all those reminders into a memory box (that you promise yourself not to open for at least a year) and lock it away. If you know the box is somewhere in your home, even if it's locked up, you might cave in and revisit these reminders. So, if you do not trust that you won't cave in, lock up this box of reminders and give the key to a friend or family member, or give the box to someone you trust to put it in their basement or attic. If you are still living with your ex, you need to permanently remove yourself from the shared space as soon as possible, or your ex needs to move out. Once you have your own space away from your ex, then you can continue with the analog detox.

Second, I'd like to introduce the "digital detox." This includes removing your ex, their friends, and your mutual contacts from all social media:

- Unfollow them and block them so they can't follow you.
- Unfollow any mutual friends, and don't let them follow you.
- No active messaging, commenting, and so on.
- Avoid passive stalking.
- Ask your friends and family to unfollow them.

Why do I recommend removing mutual contacts? You need to sort out all your current relationships into two categories: (1) who will remind you of your ex, and (2) who will help you move forward. This has nothing to do with a mutual friend being a wonderful human being or having been there for you but rather putting up healthy boundaries so you can protect yourself from your narcissistic ex. You can only do that by literally removing *all* things and people that connect you to your ex in any way whatsoever. Right now, you *need* to detox from anyone who holds any ties to your ex for your own sake, and you don't want any of your ex's life updates reaching you, or vice versa. When you have people connecting you to your ex who you truly care about, inform them of the step you're about to take and explain why you're doing it. If they are a true friend, they will more than understand and support you. If they contact you regardless, do not react to it for the time being. You can go back to adding these people to your life once you are fully over your ex. Most of the time, you won't feel the need then.

I know this is hard, but channel that rage and anger and block your ex. It gives you a sense of security that they are no longer able to reach you. *This is difficult, but remember, it's not something you're doing against your ex; it's something you're doing for yourself.* You are protecting yourself from the possibility of receiving a manipulative (sweet or sour) text or call, especially when you are lonely and vulnerable. You are protecting yourself from the masks they might put on. Blocking your ex gives you more of a chance to heal through the distance it creates. I know that blocking them will not keep a narc from contacting you (via an unknown number, a different number, a friend's phone; showing up at your house, at your work, at your favorite restaurant, at your mom's . . . the list goes on). It's not an absolute security, but it's the first step in taking back control over your life.

As I stated in the no-contact rule, the only reason to keep your ex's number in your phone is if you share children with them. How do you do keep their number in your phone but resist the urge to contact them? Start by changing their contact's name from that cute nickname with a heart to something that reminds you that you shouldn't be in contact. My personal favorite suggestion is "Do Not Answer." Further viable options are "Narc Ex," "Don't Bother," and "Not Worth It." Change it to anything that will help you resist calling them, texting them, or answering them. It may feel immature, but it works.

The next thing I suggest is taking your message history and saving that to your computer while deleting it on your phone. The point of this is to eliminate the possibility of impulsively scrolling through old messages on your phone when you are missing them. Revisiting old times only brings more pain and is never helpful. Even if you read through fights, it weirdly does not truly help you feel better. Any tie with them will pull you down, even if it's a negative one. Instead of reading through your message history, read the hate list you wrote. If you need any reminding of something, it should be a reminder of why the relationship *didn't* work out and that you deserve better!

I also recommend changing your profile picture to one where you look glowing and powerful, or something that holds special meaning to you, like a photo of your favorite pet, a flower, or a symbol. This can only make you feel better and gives you feelings of empowerment on this hard journey. It's a "fake it till you make it" thing! No subliminal messages to your ex are allowed here, no quotes about relationships, or no inside joke between the two of you.

Your phone can feel like your worst enemy—not just because it will unexpectedly show you photo memories of last Valentine's Day with your ex or because your ex might call. Not just because you catch yourself wanting to dial their number or scroll through old videos. Even your usual "fun" social media distraction now serves as a negative reminder and seems to side with your narc: The algorithm feels as if it conspires against you to make you feel worse than you already do. Social media is now feeding you constant reminders of your breakup: The algorithms will only show you heartbreak quotes, depressed pictures, sad heartbreak memes, or therapists talking about narcissism (including me!). There are two ways to beat the social media algorithms: (1) Ideally you completely pause your socials until you are truly over this breakup; or (2) you keep only a handful of the accounts that make you think about narcissism or a breakup and switch up the rest of your feed by adding accounts that are geared toward powerful affirmations, success, manifestation of your dreams, positive mindset, adorable animal accounts, or anything fun that you love or that makes you smile and feel good about life!

It's not a secret that our phones listen to us, so instead of worrying about creepy Alexa or Siri, use her to your advantage. If you feed your algorithm right by saying things like "Life is great," "affirmations," "manifestation," "I love cute animals," "cute accounts," and things like that, and search those in your Insta feed, sooner or later your phone will start showing you more of those things in your feed instead of reminding you of how horrible it is to be single right now. If it doesn't do that, don't stop to watch sad content; unfollow all your "depression" accounts. You can always pause your socials for a week or two and then come back to them. That will help reset the algorithms as well.

3. rebuild

During the rebuild phase, you begin picking up the pieces of the war zone in front of you. You can slowly start putting your puzzle—and with it, yourself—back together. After the release phase settles, it's like sandy water settling in a glass, and you will feel a sense of newfound clarity. This is the time for more self-care that you actually enjoy doing. These actions aren't grand gestures but small consistent acts of nourishing and nurturing yourself after neglecting yourself for so long.

There is something magical that usually happens around this time: You will notice yourself fully and properly—that is, *truly* being present. You haven't been present in a long time. When you're with a narc, you are never fully present because half of you is always busy trying to guess their next move, manage their next mood, or prevent their next outburst. When you are not directly with them, part of you is usually mentally absent, preoccupied with keeping in touch with the narcissist, updating them, or hoping they won't cause a scene. During the breakup, a part of you dissociates in an attempt to stay afloat. Then in the rupture and release phases, you are not fully present because you are so immersed in your pain. The rebuild phase might be the first time in a long time that that you begin to notice a glimpse of true presence. This can happen in an unexpected moment of gratitude when you simply stop your morning for a second in order to listen to birds happily chirping around you. That can feel so grounding and freeing. Or it can be a moment when you are feeling annoyed at yourself and you notice, "Hey! There is no more weight of someone else leaning on me, so how I feel right now is actually solely my responsibility and I cannot blame anyone for it!" Then you take that mood and consciously change it. This will make you feel extremely thankful for being in charge of your life again, without someone else holding power over you. It is liberating to own your responsibility by being present.

Whether it's a positive moment or a moment you feel annoyed with yourself, it doesn't matter—each is a wonderful sign of heading in the right direction!

Now is the time to counteract your identity erosion by exploring your new self without the narcissist. You are creating this new version of you that you haven't met. You will explore your passions, hobbies, and boundaries. It is key here to stay curious about every step, wondering, "What wonderful new thing in life can meet me behind this door?" rather than worrying about what bad things can happen. It is about a shift in perspective from mistrusting to being curious. Perhaps you start old hobbies again that you had to neglect because of your ex, or you learn to simply enjoy your own company. (The biggest gift, ever!) It is a slow and steady process, but within it you will learn to trust yourself again and feel safe within your skin. Again, therapy can help facilitate healing.

Each step is a step forward! In taking these steps, you could discover that you are no longer your old self, and that is absolutely okay! *The goal isn't to return to the person you were before the relationship but rather to build up a whole new, wiser, purer, more beautiful, and more authentic version of yourself.* You are now much more in tune with your own needs, so by definition you could not return to an old version of yourself. This time is not all happy, of course. It consists of much trial and error and moments of self-doubt mixed with manic outbursts of empowerment. Think of this phase as the base to build on, laying the bricks of your new life, one intentional choice at a time.

I'd like you to imagine yourself as a broken mirror. Each piece represents a part of you that has been broken by your ex. During your healing journey, you've been slowly gathering those pieces, hoping to rebuild it to look exactly like the reflection of the person you once were. But here's the bittersweet truth: Even when you manage to piece it all together, this specific mirror's reflection will never be the old you again. It is not the same. It cannot be the same, as you are no longer the same. You are a new person. Some parts of the old mirror (of your old self) are still wonderful, and others will feel like they no longer fit. There seem to be so many cracks within the glass, and its broken reflection might make you sad at first. But with time, patience, and effort, you will be able to fill those cracks with the new version of yourself and make a much more beautiful mirror—a stronger one, a wiser one, simply a gorgeous one. This mirror is one of a kind. It's a unique piece, handmade with lots of tears and sweat. It may be hard, and it may take lots of time and effort to fill up those broken parts, but one day you will be able to. Then you will see your new self clearly and with no cracks.

CHECK-IN

Write a list of the qualities or values you want included in the new reflection of your truly one-of-a-kind mirror. Make sure these are the values that are personal and authentic to you. No one else gets a say. This is all you.

The following are the top rebuild resolutions I suggest to my clients.

MEDITATION

While you were with your ex, you were not able to focus on yourself, and with that, not able to regulate your emotions. The narcissist kept you from yourself, forcing you to focus purely on them. Now that you are allowing yourself to be present for the first time, you can fully benefit from meditating. Before this phase, something like meditation—where you essentially solely focus on yourself—may have felt overwhelming and evoked feelings of anxiety. But now you can experience meditation's full benefits. You will be able to focus on your breath or a guiding voice without it causing you anxiety or any other uncomfortable "I cannot do this" feelings. You will feel a new sense of calm, be more in touch with yourself, and be more conscious of what is going on within your body. This may help you reconnect to and appreciate your body more. It may subconsciously add more feelings of gratitude to your life too.

You can practice meditation by yourself, join a meditation group, go on a retreat, do it with a friend or a family member, listen to a recording, or even practice with your therapist. You can download meditations through meditation apps or by accessing them for free on YouTube. There are different types of meditations available: self-love, body scans, cord cutting, mindfulness, visualizations on how to feel empowered, and so much more. Try them all and see which one suits you best.

(RE-)LEARN TO LEAN ON YOUR SUPPORT SYSTEM

The health of your relationships might be the most important aspect during this time, and this includes the relationship you have with yourself. If you can, surround yourself with supportive people, trusted friends, family, or a therapist who can provide support, perspective, and encouragement as you move forward. This will increase oxytocin in a healthy way as you learn to trust again. Your self-esteem will increase when you feel connected to others, further giving you a sense of self-worth, leading you away from the possibility of returning to your narc. Your fear of rejection can be a limiting factor when you think about reconnecting with friends and family you have turned your back on. That thought is valid but not always true. If your fears are partially reinforced by people refusing to reconnect, that is okay. Please accept their boundaries and turn to others who take you back with open arms. One of the greatest hockey players of all time, Wayne Gretzky, once said "You miss 100 percent of the shots you don't take." Use this wisdom and apply it! Be open to new things, even if you are unsure or scared. The point is to keep an open mind, because you never know what door may open for you next. So that next dinner or party you get invited to, go! If you do not try, you will never know. Wonderful new friendships can evolve in places you least expect. Any activity away from your ex that makes you feel alive, even for ten minutes, is a blessing and a safe base.

4. rise

The rise phase is the time where you will catch yourself having a bit of fun again for the first time in a while. It is the time where you will feel strong again and self-determined, but this is something you actively have to choose to work on, even on hard days. You will start feeling your own strength from within because of the responsibility you are now taking for your life. You might feel like an "adultier" adult, making your own decisions, not putting up with BS anymore, having erased toxic people from your life and gained clarity to know that you deserve better. All of that will fuel your power from within and help you grow in the right direction. I'm not saying everything will feel great, but an underlying pride will start to grow within you knowing you have survived so much and kept going. *You put in the work. You are the reason you're now smiling. No one else walked these steps for you, no one else completed the phases. All the credit goes to you.* That is a newfound sense of power.

In the meantime, your focus will slowly but surely shift from dwelling on the past to cautiously considering the future. You haven't been able to even contemplate the future because you were so caught up with your ex. Now it might not all be clear, but you will allow room for possibilities to unfold. In short, you'll give life the opportunity to surprise you. Remember that growth, just like healing, isn't linear. You will face setbacks, doubts, and frustrations. The difference is that you are better equipped to handle them in a mature manner now. This doesn't mean that you're immune to fear or pain but rather you now know how to navigate through them without losing yourself or being consumed.

Sometimes owning control of your life means making tough choices, such as cutting ties, setting strict boundaries, and changing old habits that you once clung to. But it will all be worth it when you see yourself coming together again. You're moving forward, one step at a time.

Mia's Story

"I did the work. I didn't place all the blame on my ex. I will never stop doing the work because no matter what, my children are always watching me. I want them to have a childhood they don't have to heal from. We were married for four years and have two children together. I celebrate and reframe these anniversaries as the days I chose my children without knowing it. I never have said, 'I wish I never met this person,' and instead thank him for the greatest blessings and lessons of my life."

The following are the top rise resolutions I suggest to my clients.

GRATITUDE JOURNAL

The rise phase is something to be proud of! No day is perfect, and there will be setbacks, but there is no reason to allow those days to bring you down. That is why having a gratitude journal is a little reminder you have for yourself of all the pain and suffering you pushed through and are now on the other side of. You do not need to do this every day, but by writing in a gratitude journal, you reflect on all your positive achievements, things you are grateful for, the simple pleasures in life, as well as track your growth and progress. Using a gratitude journal can help shift your focus from challenges to positive aspects of your life. It is time to be your life's biggest cheerleader!

DON'T GET MAD, GET PAID

As I mentioned earlier, turn the pain, the trauma, the suffering into power—into money! Remind yourself of the passions or hobbies that the narc used to belittle and criticize you and get back into them. Prove to yourself that the narc was wrong! You *are* good at (*fill in the blank*). Even better, why not try making money from it? There's no greater feeling than turning your pain into profit, gaining from your struggle rather than letting it hold you down. If you're an artist, paint your emotions and sell your artwork! If you're an athlete, train harder than ever before and use that strength to win competitions or become a coach. If you love being a parent, embrace it wholeheartedly and build a community around it, such as a blog or social media page to help those who are co-parenting with a narc partner. You can even write your own book talking about your experience with a narcissistic partner. Imagine how much it can help others, and you get paid. The point is, you never know what can come out of pursuing your passions or hobbies, so gain from your pain.

CELEBRATE ALL YOUR SMALL VICTORIES

After an eternity of being belittled and devalued by your ex, you deserve the opposite. Who better to take responsibility for making you feel good about yourself than you? It is your job, and your job only, to validate, love and take care of yourself by taking back autonomy and responsibility for your healing. Even if you don't feel it, fake it till you make it.

Healing consists of a series of small steps forward. Pause here to celebrate after every single one of those small steps you take. Acknowledging your steps will give you back control and make you feel much stronger in the process. I know this can be hard, given the history with your narc, but you need to view this as your way of investing in your well-being. Celebrating these mini victories will feel very right after a while, without feeling silly. Eventually this practice will increase your dopamine in a healthy way, just like a gratitude list for minor things you're thankful for.

Your art of celebration can be very personal and doesn't have to please anyone else. Celebrating a successful step for you could mean treating yourself to a quiet moment in a bathtub or a walk with your pet. It doesn't have to be a grand celebration, and it definitely doesn't have to be public. Unless you want to go all out, then feel free to enjoy it! Do whatever feels authentic to you, and make it personal. I like to think of it as being self-compassionate, practicing kindness toward yourself just like you would do for others. You are healing from a narcissistic abuse relationship and that is difficult enough as is, so every step away from that relationship geared toward healing is worth acknowledging. It doesn't mean you're an imposter or exaggerate your victories; it simply means you're choosing resilience. *Showing up for yourself by being kind is not indulgent, it's necessary.*

Ada's Story
"*After I realized I have to put myself first, I knew I was the only one holding the power to improve my life. As I started fitness, dance, and foreign language classes, I noticed that others began to see the resilience in me, and that recognition motivated me to keep going. Over time, I could see change within myself in the mirror: my face, my mood—all of it changed for the better. I began to appreciate the simple things and enjoy what I have. Usually I celebrated with my family, going out with friends on trips, or making gifts to myself like spa days and relaxing treatments. I realized doing things I enjoyed helped me heal from within.*"

5. radiance

The radiance phase is the last phase of grieving a narc breakup. This is where peace and self-love settle within you. This inner light stems from all the hard work you have put in that slowly taught you to trust yourself again. You have taken your life back into your own hands and are now able to proudly show the scars from the pain that shaped you. You are no longer embarrassed for them but rather proud of them. You feel stronger, as described in Christina Aguilera's "Fighter."

All the relationships you now have, including the new one you have with yourself, begin to feel healthier. You are no longer surrounded by toxicity or people taking advantage of your kind heart, and you are not allowing anyone to abuse you. You know what you want and need, and you will not settle for less than you deserve. *Knowing that people can only use you if you let them is no longer a scary thought but a calming one now.*

You most likely feel clarity and a sense of bliss. Both were hard-earned as you put in the work, and it is now showing in the way you carry yourself. You are no longer running away from your past. You are now happy to be in your present as well as walking toward the future of your own making. You're living with more intention and a heartfelt purpose.

Moments of vulnerability feel like old friends are visiting. They do not scare you or make you weak. You handle those moments with grace and compassion for your inner child, not letting them control you. Your once small and tight world with the narc feels very open and rich again—not because you are guaranteed a smooth ride but because you know that whatever life throws at you, you will make the right decision on how to engage and handle it. You are simply ready for what life has in store for you, and you trust the universal alignment.

The following are the top radiance resolutions I suggest to my clients.

EXPLORE NEW ACTIVITIES

Choose some activity that genuinely gets you going. Join a hip-hop dance class, a pottery course, a new hiking or running club—whatever feels right with your newfound self. Start small, but commit to it. Don't make plans for something that will take up five days of your week and then toss it after two weeks, as that always feels like a failure to keep your promises to yourself. Perhaps choose something less time consuming in the beginning that you can then expand on if you fully fall in love with it, the people in it, or the feelings you get out of it.

In the beginning, you might feel a bit out of place or even ridiculous with your newfound hobby—that's to be expected when trying something new! Don't let that stop you from doing it, and know that growth often requires discomfort. You will be so proud of yourself if you withstand those feelings of irritation in the beginning and dive into a whole new world. Also, don't forget that it is not about perfecting something, such as learning to play the guitar like Carlos Santana, but rather enjoying yourself and gifting yourself a beautiful time doing something positive and creative. There is also something very positive about connecting to other people who mean well and love the same things you do. It's simply a chance to build new friendships or more! Putting yourself out there and trying new stuff should be celebrated! Acknowledge your courage for leaving your fears behind and not letting them hold you back.

MAKE A BUCKET LIST

Now that you're completely free and disconnected from your ex, the real fun can begin with no strings attached! One of my favorite things to do for myself, and something I highly recommend to clients, is creating a bucket list for your near future that you can actually check off! Make it achievable and fun. Why not? Take all the things you've thought about trying, exploring, and experiencing. A personal bucket list can range from something as simple and easily achievable as going to the movies alone, all the way to something extravagant and maybe even complicated such as traveling to South America by yourself to explore the Amazon. A nice rule of thumb is to create a bucket list of ten items with at least six of them being easily achievable so that you don't have to wait for next year's Christmas bonus or your next milestone birthday to bring your ideas to life.

My experience has shown me that if you follow these resolutions, you are guaranteed to be heading in the right direction. Of course, they do not all need to be taken at once or in the exact order of the book, but they do need to be followed at some point. When you apply all of them at your own pace, you will find peace on your path through every single step, understanding that they have been created to guide you back to yourself. No one said this will be easy; in fact, it will be really hard. There will be times when you want to quit, when you feel like giving up is the easier option. That might be true, but just because it's easy doesn't mean it's right.

Choose what is right over what is easy. Choose yourself and your heart's healing.

To my clients, I always say that when you choose yourself over a narcissist, the most important thing to keep in mind is that *you have to put your mind over your heart*. Your mind knows why you are leaving the narc. Your mind knows and understands that this is right for you and that you deserve better. Your heart often doesn't know it *yet*. Like jet lag, your heart still needs time to be convinced, as a heart's job is to cling to the love and hope you feel in hard times. A heart's job is to love unconditionally, while your mind's job is to protect you from people who don't deserve that love. So, view it as a jet lag of the heart and soul, and give your heart some time to reach the place your mind is already at. This will help you stick to doing the right thing—leaving them and loving yourself. You are done with doing the wrong thing—staying with them/taking them back and accepting their malicious treatment.

This journey to the new you is not a quick fix, and it takes time. It may take you months, a year, or several years to reach this point of fully moving on. This does not just come on its own; it requires patience and commitment. Channel your pain, suffering, and determination to be free and turn them into a source of strength. *Remember: The goal is to stay free and never go back to another toxic relationship.*

ONE LAST REMINDER

They lost you, and you lost nothing! What you thought they were doesn't exist, but you do. Everything you made them out to be was your belief in their potential (your projections) and your hope that they would again be the person they once were (their facade that you believed in). They are none of that; it was all your generosity and love. Leaving them means that you are now free from the toxic dynamic of this twisted relationship that never served you. You are now given the opportunity for a greater life and a love that is actually real—the love for yourself. Take it!

part four

staying free

chapter 10

coping tools after the breakup

"We repeat what we don't repair."

—Christine Langley-Obaugh

In the previous chapters, I have mentioned coping tools to use during your relationship with a narc in order to manage your situation. Now that you have left them, please continue to use those tools, as well as the new tools I am about to introduce to you. These new tools are specifically useful to give you the power to stay free from the narc from now on. It all starts with you and your own reflection.

reflection

You're probably asking yourself, "Now that I am away, how do I ensure that I do not get involved with another narc?" The first thing you need to do, now that some time has passed and the dust has settled, is reflect on what happened. You need to reflect while being brutally honest with yourself in order to heal and put the pieces back together.

Ask yourself the hard questions, put up boundaries, learn to say no, and challenge yourself. In *My Toxic Breakup: A Guided Journal*, I guide you through some of the most important questions you need to ask. Write them down and answer them for yourself before you do anything else. Here are three I find very helpful to begin with.

1. What was my contribution to the toxicity?
2. Why did I choose to be with my ex in the first place?
3. What was is that made me miss or ignore all the red flags with my ex?

This reflection is essential. It is the foundation on which you can build from now on. It's important to identify your role in the relationship, not because you are to blame but to understand how you contributed to the dynamic, why you chose someone with toxic behaviors, and how you may have ignored the signs. This is all part of growing and healing. Once you understand what the consequences of your answers mean for you, you are ready to dive into your toolbox further and continue your journey.

group therapy

Group therapy is a great way to gain support and connection with others who have gone through emotional abuse from a narcissist. You will hear similar experiences, and this will remind you that you are not alone with this pain. Getting support from other survivors is invaluable, as they truly understand you. You are not invisible to them. They see you and they see your pain, just like you see theirs. Group therapy can improve self-efficacy and decrease depression, so it is an important resource. Through successful group therapy, you will be able to rebuild your trust in others, possibly find new friends, facilitate mutual healing, and feel less isolated through the safe space of sharing experiences together. Also, the once-a-week setting gives you routine and safety.

I want to take a moment to warn you about some potential disadvantages of group therapy, as I've found that certain clients may not fully benefit. Group therapy is not a fit for all. There is the possibility of an emotional overload when you hear others' stories and that can be retraumatizing. Though sharing is essential for healing, the weight of their trauma might leave you exhausted after sessions. Further, I personally don't like the dynamic of comparison and competition that often arises in a group therapy setting. Sometimes members unintentionally fall into the trap of comparing trauma and make others feel undermined in their own experience as someone else's story seems "so much worse." This often leads to invalidation of personal pain. When a member feels like their own experience is insignificant, they often withdraw and feel more isolated than before, fueling their feelings of inadequacy.

However, do not let this discourage you from trying group therapy to see how you feel about it. Everyone is different, and some people are not affected by these dynamics. A lot also depends on the leader of the group. With a lot of experience, the leader will see the ruptures and competition within the group dynamic and address it. If you experience the possible pitfalls of group therapy, know that it's not your fault, it's not the weight of your story, and it's not you. It's just a group dynamic that isn't your fit! Try another group.

If you are unable to attend in-person group therapy, consider exploring online options such as virtual support groups or therapy apps. There are wonderful websites for online support that provide judgment-free environments. I give you my favorites in the resource section. These specialized survivor forums offer flexible and safe environments to connect with others who share similar experiences. These spaces can provide support and validation, ensuring you don't feel isolated during your healing journey.

self-care and nurturing

Alongside therapy, self-care is fundamental in your recovery. It can be something very simple and private you do for yourself or something social and connected. Conscious self-care will naturally restore your cortisol levels, heighten your mood, and act as your body's natural painkiller. Here are some of my personal favorites:

Maintain a consistent sleep schedule. Adequate and consistent sleep is essential for your brain and body. When you get enough rest, you are better able to make decisions, problem-solve, and maintain attention and focus, all of which contribute to healing.

Spend time with loved ones. Do things with them that fill your cup: crafting, baking cookies, playing interactive video games . . . anything that makes you happy. Don't only spend it on talking about your ex!

Make food your religion. Your body has been through a lot, and you only have one! Be kind to yourself by cooking healthy meals and eating consciously. Eat at regular intervals, and make sure you get three healthy meals a day. Avoid overeating.

Practice mindful eating. When you eat, make sure you do nothing but eat. No cell phone, laptop, playing with your cat. Just focus on eating. This will increase your gratitude for the food and make you eat slower and more consciously.

Put away your phone. When you walk—by yourself or with your pet—walk without the phone. Ensure your focus is purely on the nature around you. When you meet a friend, put your phone on silent and put it away. Just be there consciously with your friend. See if that makes a difference in your connection! Make it a habit to turn off your phone after 6 p.m. Put away your phone at night, pause socials, and silence notifications—anything you can do to clear some space in your mind. Doing a twenty-four-hour or weekend digital detox will also have a positive impact. No matter what you do, do one thing at a time, without checking your phone or responding to messages. Allow awareness to settle in and calm you down.

Take a warm bath or a nice long shower. Pamper yourself with a little massage, body lotion, a face mask, or a special hair product. Anything good for your body and beauty is good for your mind.

Read self-help books that can unlock your healing potential. Here are my personal favorites that really impacted my life and perspective:

- *Happier: Learn the Secrets to Daily Joy and Lasting Fulfillment* by Tal Ben-Shahar

- *Radical Acceptance: Embracing Your Life with the Heart of a Buddha* by Tara Brach

- *Solve for Happy: Engineer Your Path to Joy* by Mo Gawdat

- *The Happiness Code: 10 Keys to Being the Best You Can Be* by Domonique Bertolucci

- *The Millionaire and the Monk: A True Story about the Meaning of Life* by Julian Hermsen

- *The Miracle Morning: The Not-So-Obvious Secret Guaranteed to Transform Your Life (Before 8 a.m.)* by Hal Elrod

- *The Untethered Soul: The Journey Beyond Yourself* by Michael A. Singer

- *Whole Again: Healing Your Heart and Rediscovering Your True Self after Toxic Relationships and Emotional Abuse* by Jackson MacKenzie

Volunteer. I loved volunteering at animal shelters, but whatever floats your boat is best. There are shelters for the homeless where you can help serve food or talk to people and listen to their stories. You can volunteer at hospitals, elderly homes, food pantries, and schools. Take up a cause and get involved in related activities. Volunteer work can be immensely enriching because you get back so much more than you put in.

Find some mentors. One of my good friends, Sumair Greene, shares his go-to approach that I love: Focus on five mentors. "Keep your inner circle small, and choose those few wisely!" He advises picking five mentors you truly admire and immersing yourself in their work—read every book they've written, listen to their podcasts, watch their shows, and follow them closely on social media. Leave everyone else out. This streamlined approach might be the fastest path to healing. I agree with him on this and thought it was an idea worth sharing. You'll be better off focusing on a single path rather than following conflicting advice from many. So, choose your circle wisely, commit to it, and let their wisdom guide your journey.

Listen to great music. I am obsessed with music and couldn't get through one day without it. I think music is absolutely essential for healing. Whether you relax to good jazz, dance to hip-hop, or scream with heavy metal, let your emotions have some space and express them through good music.

Pamper yourself. Get a haircut, barber shave, manicure, pedicure, facial, or massage; go to a steam room or sauna. Even retail therapy in moderation can do wonders for your self-esteem. Treat yourself to something you love, something that makes you feel good. Remember, you are worth it!

> ### CHECK-IN
>
> *Try your very own thirty-day self-care commitment challenge. Choose one nurturing practice each day. Whether it's a warm bath, digital detox, or a mindful meal, commit to the practice for a month and notice the shifts in your emotional well-being.*

release rituals

Release rituals are seemingly counterintuitive to practicing breathwork and meditation, but combining the two is like a yin-and-yang practice for your wounded soul. Breathwork and meditation focus on calming your mind and body, just like the yin concept represents the feminine, passive, and receptive energies that are soft and nurturing. Release rituals allow your mind and body to release all the pent-up pain, suffering, and tension in a cathartic way, just like the yang concept represents the masculine, active, and assertive energies within you. Such outward action is energetic and strong. I like thinking of the two as complementary rather than opposing forces. This duality means you can live with both sides of yourself, without holding any guilt or shame. One side cannot exist without the other, and you do not have to choose between them. They can work together to bring balance to your inner world. You have been abused, and it hurts. The pain is there to remind you not to engage with your abuser or continue the relationship. The pain is your friend; don't try to silence it.

high-adrenaline sports

High-adrenaline sports is one of the best ways to let out pent-up anger and pain without thinking about it. Releasing negative emotions can even enhance your performance. You can use them to your advantage. My personal favorites are:

- Agility training with a dog (Train with your own or work with a shelter/rescue dog! They will be so grateful!)
- Boxing
- CrossFit

- HIIT
- Horse polo
- Muay Thai
- Running
- Skydiving
- Water sports

non-adrenaline activities

Though they are more meditative than high-adrenaline sports, non-adrenaline activities will also help you release your emotions. They can feel slow and beautiful and still let feelings flow out just as effectively.

- Baking
- Dancing
- Flow writing

- Gardening
- Hot yoga
- Vision jar

All these release rituals are especially beneficial to survivors. Due to the intense concentration these activities require, your body reaches a state of flow. In this state, you are releasing everything toxic from your past. It's a cleansing of mind and body that leaves you feeling powerful.

words of affirmation

When you are kind to yourself, you feel better about yourself. Stand in front of a mirror and look at yourself with love, compassion, and kindness and say these five affirmations:

1. I am worthy of love and respect.
2. I am learning and growing from this experience.
3. I am free to create the life I want.
4. I am in control of my own happiness.
5. I accept and love myself unconditionally.

If you don't feel ready for these affirmations, try the following, according to the stage of your healing.

Early stage
- I am in the process of healing, and that is enough.
- I am learning to love and trust myself, one step at a time.
- I forgive myself for the past and allow myself to move forward.

Middle stage
- I am growing stronger and more resilient every day.
- I am worthy of love, respect, and kindness.
- I choose to honor my boundaries and prioritize my well-being.

Later stage
- I am whole, complete, and ready to welcome healthy connections.
- I am capable of creating a life filled with joy and purpose.
- I trust myself to make decisions that reflect my self-worth.

journaling

Another powerful way to practice self-care is through journaling, and I highly recommend it. Writing down your thoughts and feelings is incredibly therapeutic, helping you process and reflect on your emotions while bringing greater clarity. Channeling your emotions through writing allows you to release them on paper. Imagine your thoughts like a river running through you. If you let them out—by journaling, acting, screaming, singing, drawing, and so forth—the water (thoughts) just runs through you and therefore has no power to hurt you. If you don't let it out, let it run through you, it's like putting up a dam, and the dam will trap your anxiety, fear, and anger inside. When you let water (thoughts) simply pass through you, balance can return naturally. The emotions flow freely, they no longer have a grip on you, and you can experience clarity and freedom.

The great thing about journaling is that your journal will not judge you. Your journal will not make you feel bad. Your journal will not hurt you. Write it all out—no filter. Over time, you can refer to these journal entries to help remind you of everything you've experienced and survived. It will remind you of your strength in times of doubt.

I believe so much in the therapeutic and healing benefits of journaling that I've created a thirty-day guided journal called My Toxic Breakup: A Guided Journal, designed to help you navigate a breakup from a toxic relationship. Find it in the resource section.

CHECK-IN

Journaling prompt: What emotion am I ready to release today? What would it feel like to let it go?

---

forgiveness and letting go

To truly move forward, forgiveness is key: forgiveness toward your abuser (this does not mean ever going back to your abuser!), forgiveness toward anyone who did not believe or support you during or after the relationship, and forgiveness toward yourself—for loving them, for staying, and for feeling raw now.

The idea of forgiveness is easier said than done, but it is essential to let go of the weight of the abuse, shame, guilt, and betrayal so you can move forward. In psychology, acceptance is a key part of therapy. An immensely powerful practice is "radical acceptance." It means to accept everything as it is, without wanting to change it. I encourage you to accept everything that has happened, accept everything that is currently happening, and accept the unknown of the future. Accepting reality for what it is reduces your pain and fear and improves your ability to cope and move on. Once you accept it all, forgiveness has a safe place to settle in. All you need to do is work on accepting what is and not fight it. The rest will follow if you are continuously patient and kind with yourself.

Often we are stuck in the denial stage or bargaining stage of grief. That is more than understandable, but without accepting what is, there is no way forward. Acceptance is not a one-and-done practice but a lifelong commitment. There will always be things that are difficult around or inside us, and radically accepting them frees up the soul. Whenever you get a chance, sit with your negative thoughts or feelings and practice a two-minute radical acceptance mediation.

radical acceptance practice

Here is a two-minute radical acceptance meditation you can practice daily:

- Get in a comfortable position and close your eyes.

- Take a deep breath in through your nose, and slowly exhale through your mouth. Feel your body relax as you release tension with each breath.

- Now bring your awareness to whatever you are feeling in this moment— whether it's peace, discomfort, anxiety, or sadness. Simply notice it, without trying to change or judge it. Just allow it to be.

- Continue to breathe and silently say to yourself, "This is how it is right now."

- Allow yourself to acknowledge the present, accepting whatever arises. Remember, acceptance doesn't mean approval. It's simply the act of being with what is, without resistance. If difficult emotions come up, offer them compassion. Picture yourself embracing those feelings with kindness, like you would comfort a close friend.

- Breathe in acceptance, and breathe out judgment.

- On your next breath, silently say, "I am here, and everything is okay." Let the truth of this settle in. Stay with your breath, knowing that whatever you're feeling or facing, you have the capacity to meet it with gentleness.

- Take one more deep breath in, and slowly exhale. When you're ready, gently open your eyes.

Once you feel comfortable with practicing radical acceptance, you can also try active forgiveness, the next step toward inner peace.

active forgiveness

This is done by following four important steps:

1. Acknowledge what happened to you, the things you allowed the narc to get away with and the lessons you had to learn. Reflect on each and every one of those moments and write them down. It's okay to relive the emotions. I know they are painful, but ignoring or trying to bury them deep down is not the answer. Let the wounds have the space that they deserve.

2. Understand the context. Remind yourself that you were controlled and manipulated and that this could have happened to anyone. You did not actively choose wrong; you were wronged. There is a big difference. Knowing the context and all their tactics and masks is vital for reaching some self-love and understanding. Simply accept the responsibility of what happened to you as yours in order to let it go.

3. Practice the same compassion you would offer a close friend. It is common to have feelings of shame, guilt, or embarrassment for being so naive and falling for the narc's lies. Still, this is the moment for the opposite of self-loathing. It's the moment for compassion. Consider if your closest friend had gone through what you did. How would you be there for them if they told you they're so stupid and ashamed of themselves for being where they are right now? You would offer them love and try to lift them up by reminding them of who they are! You would be kind, patient, and warmhearted. Why be different to yourself? Be your own best friend and give yourself the compassion you deserve! Apologize to yourself for not protecting yourself better and promise that you will do so in the future.

4. Learn from the experience. By educating yourself on the topic, like reading this book and following its suggestions, you are doing everything you can to not fall for a narc trap again. View it as a huge gain and place it in your toolbox as a lesson learned. If you ever need it in the future, you know where to look! This will ensure you make better choices in your future and choose new partners wisely.

Accept every part of your journey and celebrate your successes without fear of backsliding, as that is part of the process. You can harness all your energy toward building a brighter future for yourself.

Afet's Story

"Yoga, meditation, and therapy increased my awareness. Maybe if I had not experienced this pain, I would not have gained this awareness. Being aware—most importantly, being aware of myself—is important to wake up. I was burned inside more than I have ever felt in my life, my heart ached, and my pride was broken, but I chose to rise from the ashes."

spiritual rituals during a full moon

For those of you who are spiritual, there is one more thing that can feel very cleansing. I call it a "full moon ritual à la Maria" (my wonderful spiritual teacher and friend). Use every full moon to do the following three things:

1. Write a list of things you want to let go of. Simply sit down and write a list of things that no longer serve you in your life or things you want to get rid of (e.g., fear of the unknown, being lazy in the mornings, and so on). Once you have your list written, go to a safe place in your house or outside and burn this piece of paper, thereby releasing their hold on you.

2. Write a list of things you want to manifest in your life. Keep the list of manifestations in a safe place to look at frequently; do not destroy it.

3. Cleanse your home with white sage. For those who believe in smoking out energies to clear up your space, you can burn white sage bundles and walk through your entire home, staying a bit longer in places that are important to you (such as your bed, your desk, your couch, your baby's crib). Then, after you have smoked up your place, open all the windows for fifteen minutes and let the energies clear out. White sage is believed to bundle up old energies, and opening the windows will take all of them outside.

These three things during a full moon will leave you empowered and connected to your inner spirit warrior. It feels nice and empowering to restart each month with the moon phases.

As we come to the end of this chapter, take a moment to honor the courage it has taken to break free and stay free! All the investment you've made. All your energy. All your time. You've equipped yourself with tools to protect your peace and nurture your growth beyond the ordinary. No matter how small, each choice you make to care for yourself, seek support, and embrace your healing journey is a declaration of your worth. You are no longer bound by the past or your toxic ex. You are actively creating a future filled with strength, joy, and freedom! I am very proud of you.

chapter 11

moving forward: rising in love with yourself

"You yourself, as much as anybody in the entire universe, deserves your love and affection."

—Buddha

For some of you, depending on how quickly you finished this book, meeting a new partner might feel extremely far away right now, but dating is just around the corner of healing! Because you are still a bit fragile, it's important to follow a few rules.

dating yourself first

Before dating others, it's important to start by dating yourself. You don't have to wait—start today. You're laughing at me right now? Don't! I mean it!

My suggestion might sound quite unusual, but treating yourself as you would treat a new flame is incredibly rewarding! This phase is not about waiting around until you are ready to date other people; rather, it's about finding joy in your own company and filling up your cup before sharing it with anyone. This phase is truly sacred.

Why should you date yourself first? Dating yourself lets you rebuild a sense of self-worth. It's a period in your life where you fully focus on you and don't fall back into toxic patterns with future partners. It gives you the chance to start loving your own company. You may rediscover this ability of being on your own and enjoying life without a partner, or it may be the first time you experience this infectious, liberating feeling! Ultimately, dating yourself and enjoying your own company is a gift that no one can take away from you. It's yours. You will be able to fully enjoy your "me time" rather than worry about being alone. It helps you prioritize your healing by protecting your emotional well-being because no one else is allowed into your sacred space for now. You are the boss and get to decide for how long that space is a no-go zone for other people.

Start by exploring your needs and desires. Maybe you try a niche activity that your ex would have judged you for, or something your ex considered lame, such as crochet. Whatever it is, find out what actually floats your boat by trying new things. You never know if you don't try. Sometimes things are different in our head than they are in real life. Maybe you always wanted to try bouldering, but once you did, you realized it's not your thing. That's absolutely fine, because now you know. Maybe another activity your friend drags you to turns out to become your favorite hobby. Either way, explore and enjoy yourself while trying new things.

In addition, take yourself on dates. Watch the sun set or rise with your pet, go see a great film, get coffee at your favorite bookstore or café, check out a museum, or go on a picnic and bring a good book. These things cost virtually nothing, and you don't need a partner to enjoy them. If you are feeling comfortable with the idea, and you are having fun dating yourself, I also suggest a slightly deeper ritual, such as planning a solo getaway for yourself or dedicating a specific day each week to an activity that brings you (and only you!) joy. This will reinforce the idea of self-sufficiency and self-love every week and deepen your experience with this practice.

CHECK-IN

After you have spent some time with yourself, ask yourself these questions:

> *What dates with myself make me feel truly alive and happy?*
>
> *How has spending time alone changed my perspective on being single?*
>
> *How has it changed my perspective on relationships?*
>
> *How has this time alone raised the standards for the kinds of dates I want to be taken on?*

Once you immerse yourself in this phase, you might get addicted to spending time with yourself and the amazing feeling of pure freedom and gratitude that comes with it. Don't worry about becoming antisocial, and don't worry about staying in this phase for too long. Your body will tell you exactly when it's enough of "me, myself, and I" time and when you are ready to start meeting new people. Once you regain trust in yourself, you'll have an easier time making healthy decisions about future partners and what it is you truly want.

manifesting your ideal partner

Sometimes we can use our painful experiences to our advantage instead of constantly blaming ourselves for getting into those situations to begin with. Having been with someone toxic made me very picky. At the same time, it made the process so much more efficient as I conserved time and mental effort by not engaging with people who fell short of my list. It was excruciating to let go, because when you're in a relationship with a narcissist, your self-confidence and self-preservation instincts start to dwindle. You sometimes doubt your own sanity and question whether you just have extremely high standards. However, once you step away from the relationship for a while, you realize what a nightmare it was, and you realize that you don't want to endure more pain.

Therefore, before dating others, it is very important for you to engage in some reflection after the "me, myself, and I" phase to determine what you truly want and need in a healthy future partner. My favorite part of this journey, a very empowering one, is creating a "perfect partner" manifestation list. To do this, take out your journal and at the top of a fresh page write down "My perfect partner." Then, one by one, add all the points that you can think of that are important to you.

Kat's Story
"After ending things with my ex, I made a list of qualities I wanted in a partner, and that's how I met my current husband shortly thereafter. The list wasn't extensive, but it focused on my core values, and I wanted someone who was confident in themselves, thereby allowing me to take center stage sometimes and not compete for attention."

I want to give you several tips on creating this list so that it is a meaningful tool and not just a paper with ten words on it. When you reread this list, you should truly be touched and feel it inside you; excitement, happiness, and a sprinkle of hope and faith should arise. When that happens, you are actually manifesting all these things to come into your life. That is when you're open for change. That's when you're ready to find a new, healthy partner.

CHECK-IN

As you start to create your list, close your eyes and imagine your ideal partner. How do they make you feel? Picture the joy, safety, and connection you'll share. Allow these feelings to guide your list.

For this perfect partner to actually materialize, there are several things to keep in mind. Here is an outline for what to focus on so that your list serves you well and you get what you want. There are three important categories that you need to keep in mind: the must-haves, the nice-to-haves, and the deal-breakers. Let's start with the must-haves.

1. First, include all the must-have anti-narc qualities that are essential to you in a partner. Take time to elaborate on each quality, clearly defining what it means to you. Provide specific examples that resonate with your personal values.

   a. My favorite anti-narc qualities that you can elaborate on are: empathetic, compassionate, responsible, accountable, consistent, supportive, collaborative, kind, selfless when needed, emotionally intelligent, self-aware, and respectful. They should always be your cheerleader, believe in you when you don't believe in yourself, be a positive spirit, be a team player, put you before them, and accept and support your boundaries.

   b. For example, write down "Responsibility," and then explain what that means to you: "I want my perfect partner to be present with me and my kids rather than be on their phone all the time, to own their mistakes and apologize, to love family dinners like I love them and always prioritize this special time together without distractions, to follow through on their promises, and to organize family financials with me."

2. Now that you have essential anti-narc qualities written down, you can move on to the other must-haves as well as nice-to-haves. Be sure to include qualities that are specifically important to you in a partner. Keep the must-haves list short but precise—no more than ten.

   a. These aspects include but are not limited to views and opinions of religion, politics, animals, health, sports, vacations, family dynamics, work, free time, priorities, friendship, money, raising kids, and education.

   b. For me, an important must-have example would be my partner has to be kind to animals. He has to love them wholeheartedly, never wish them harm, and accept my dog as part of our daily family life. I would want him to take responsibility for Amari as if she were his own, if needed. I need him to not have a problem sharing tasks when I am unable to do them, such as walking her when I am sick and feeding her if I am unavailable. This is a nonnegotiable for me. On the other hand, a nice-to-have quality would be height. For me specifically, it would be nice if he were taller than me.

   c. Manifest each point that is important to you and take time to think about them, imagine them, and feel them within you. Imagine them happening as you write.

3. Once you have written down your must-haves and nice-to-haves, write down your deal-breakers. Your personal examples can be drawn from your hate list from your ex for inspiration!

   a. These aspects include but are not limited to: selfish, arrogant, manipulative, lying, triangulating, faking, devaluing, controlling, explosive, impulsive, judgmental, dramatic, stingy, vain, having a victim mentality, inconsistent, need for attention and admiration, jealous, hateful, spiteful, bad in bed, and a bad kisser! Here, again, make sure you elaborate on the specific points depending on what is truly a pet peeve for you.

b. For example, my personal biggest deal-breaker would be a man who is stingy—emotionally, spiritually, and financially. I feel these people are small in their mindset and don't allow space for big, beautiful things to unravel in their lives. They feel like no one deserves their money, their time, or their energy, which makes them entitled and unappealing for me. It is an absolute deal-breaker.

4. Now sleep on it. The next day or several days later, look at that list and cross-check for the following:

a. Was this list similar to the one you had in your head before you met your narc, and could that be dangerous? Are you looking for things that will get you into trouble (e.g., bad-boy qualities)?

b. Are you focused on too many superficial points (e.g., she needs to be fit and young) or do you have enough depth in your list?

c. Is this list realistic, or are you already avoiding meeting an ideal partner by making an impossible list (e.g., they need to be ripped, rich, gorgeous, and successful)?

setting realistic expectations

Let's be honest: You can't expect perfection in a partner. Nobody is perfect, not even you. You can't expect your partner to be superhuman. You need to show up with the same energy that you are looking for. Take the time to look inward and reflect on what you bring to the table for your future partner, then set realistic expectations on what they should bring to the table for you. If you are not satisfied with what you bring to the table, work on yourself until you are, and then start dating. Relationships are a balance of giving and receiving—a two-way street. Know your worth, understand what you offer, and seek someone who matches that in a realistic way.

Setting realistic expectations includes differentiating between must-haves, nice-to-haves, and deal-breakers. Must-haves are qualities you cannot forgo. These have to be present in your partner, and if the new person you've met does not have them, stop seeing them immediately—no excuses. Nice-to-haves are things you would like but may not always receive, and that is okay. You need to be flexible with these. Deal-breakers are just what they sound like. If your new potential partner has the qualities you hate, you need to move on immediately—again, no excuses. This part is hard and seems to reduce the possibility of finding "the one" even more. But remember, there are eight billion people in this world and you only need one "the one." It's cute to believe in potential rather than what is actually there, but remember where that got you last time—into a hellhole of pain. No more believing in potential; we are all adults and are not about to change 180 degrees. You are not sixteen anymore. This person is showing you who they are: See it, accept it, and move on to finding the right person.

When people struggle to find what they're looking for in a partner, it's often because they've set unrealistic expectations. For example, creating a thirty-point list of must-haves is setting the bar extremely high. Expecting someone to check every single box is unfair. On the flip side, some people ignore their deal-breakers entirely, which leads to settling for less than they deserve and repeating old patterns.

When you put in all this work and effort into self-reflection and your manifesting-your-dream-partner list, you will show up differently. You will show up with confidence and self-respect. You will be coming not from a place of lack but from a place of self-sufficiency and even abundance, so you will not need someone else to fill your cup. Your cup is already full of self-respect and self-love. This will ensure that your future relationships are healthy and fulfilling; otherwise, you will see no need for them.

CHECK-IN

Even with all the best intentions and a positive attitude, emotional setbacks are to be expected. Whenever you experience one, take a deep breath and pause; allow yourself to recognize any challenging feelings without judgment. Accept each emotion (radical acceptance!) and think about what you need most right now. Maybe it's rest? A comforting activity or person you love? (Not your ex!) Choose one small action to nurture yourself, even if it's just for a few minutes. Now remind yourself that setbacks are to be expected in healing. Say a simple affirmation, such as "I am moving forward, even in small steps."

avoidance behaviors to watch out for

When you reenter the dating game after being in a narcissistic relationship, you are often faced with triggers. Anyone—even healthy individuals—can remind you of your ex and/or abusive traits, create (over-)reactions inside you, or get you into overthinking. During this time, you might also find yourself engaging in avoidance behaviors. Some avoidance behaviors protect you from more harm and are useful and good to practice, but others that I will now explain can impede your healing or slow down your recovery process.

Avoidance behaviors—behaviors that distract you from your pain—often kick in post-breakup in order to alleviate painful emotions. They manifest through self-sabotage in various forms. There is no one-size-fits-all approach, as these behaviors affect everyone differently. The tricky part is that while engaging in them, you might feel they are helping you. However, this is merely the lure of instant gratification. Over the long haul, they are truly destructive, requiring more work to unlearn that far outweighs the temporary relief they provided. They will add more pain. Here are some of the most common avoidance behaviors to be aware of; be honest with yourself about whether you are engaging in them.

drinking and drugs

In a desperate attempt to numb the longing for their ex, survivors often revert to drinking and drugs, both legal and illegal. Instead, aim for long-term rewards rather than the short-term quick fix. These behaviors are simply not healthy and will not get you any closer to your goal of healing and becoming a better version of yourself. They will distract you for now and cause you problems later—potentially an addiction. If you indulge in them too much, it causes further feelings of shame and failure. If you are drinking extensively or using drugs, get help. You can't heal from abuse if you are not sober and feeling the pain. You must go through the pain in order to get out of it. No good will come from numbing it.

promiscuity

Often narc-abuse survivors start sleeping around with many people in an effort to numb their loneliness, which only leaves them feeling emptier and sadder. Choose intimate partners wisely, and make sure to use protection. Science says that our body actually connects to all people we have sex with, even if we don't mean to or consciously feel affection for them. Please protect your heart from the possible chaos, and refocus on yourself.

pushing people away

Often after a narcissistic breakup, survivors start to emotionally guard themselves by putting up walls in order to avoid getting hurt further. This might mean subconsciously rejecting genuine support from friends and family or guarding yourself from forging new relationships with new friends or possible romantic partners. This is simply another way of displaying trust issues, with yourself and others. During this time, you might subconsciously isolate yourself by canceling plans or snapping at people for no apparent reason. This can be due to feeling like a burden, a fear of vulnerability, believing others won't understand you, or feeling angry at the world for the abuse that happened to you.

You will meet many new inspiring people, and you might feel the urge to run away from them immediately, especially if it feels like another sacred connection or very strong chemistry. If you fear getting hurt and think about running in the other direction, ask yourself these questions:

- Is this person showing any of the twenty-four toxic flags?

- Do I actually mistrust this new person I met, or do I just mistrust myself and my ability to make good decisions?

- How does the fear I have about this new person actually compare to their actions? Do they align, or am I just being paranoid?

- If I separate my history from my present, am I still afraid?

- Is this new person being consistent over time?

The way you answer these questions will help determine whether you should give this person a chance. If you have a good gut feeling while answering these questions, that is a great indicator that this person is worth giving a shot. If not, then they are not the right person and you should move on. Dating again can be scary, especially when healing from trauma, but try your best to be aware, follow your lists and heart if they align, and give dating and your happiness a chance.

longing for perceived closeness

Many times, survivors fixate on memories by replaying conversations in their heads. The underlying theme is "Better to be connected through negativity than not connected at all." Although this habit can hurt the survivor, the subjective gain of "feeling closely connected" often outweighs the pain. This need to stay connected can sometimes escalate, moving from mental fixation to action. This manifests as stalking behaviors—anything that violates no-contact rules. By stalking your narcissist, you inflict emotional pain on yourself in an attempt to stay updated on their life. This creates a supposed sense of closeness. At its core, the purpose of these actions is to regain a sense of control—what psychologists often refer to as perceived control. This control is not real. The illusion of knowing their whereabouts, daily routines, and activities can provide a false sense of safety. While it may seem to ease the anxiety of uncertainty, it ultimately perpetuates your pain. Reread the section on the trauma bond and the chemical cascade in your brain so you understand what is happening and resist these temptations.

CHECK-IN

Keeping tabs on your ex only creates the illusion of control over them. It puts you back in a place where all you do is obsess over them rather than focus on yourself, making torment and anxiety within you rise, not drop. There is no point in trying to see the changes that happened after you—whether it is a new supply, a new hobby, or implementing something you always hoped for. Remember, it is in your past. Leave it there.

having a "blame brett" mentality

Have you heard the song "Blame Brett" from the Beaches? Jordan Miller sings about blaming your ex for your "f***-all" mentality. This mentality is good to a degree because you don't care about what your ex is doing—yay! But you can take it too far by turning your heart into an icebox and not caring about anyone or anything anymore. That stage is no longer "healthy moving on" but actually dwelling on pain by becoming reckless and not caring about the consequences of your actions. You went from being an empath to being coldhearted. That cannot be the solution. You can lose your job, custody of your kids, your health, your family, your resources, your identity. As a therapist, I would say that you have my full permission to feel like this, but not to act on it. There is a difference. You are a responsible adult and need to snap back into the real world if you feel yourself slipping away into this type of behavior. You want to practice kindheartedness, even if you got very hurt. You are bigger than your ex. Show it.

> ### CHECK-IN
>
> *Go through each avoidance behavior one by one and write down how it shows up for you. Then write down one action that you can take to address that behavior. This will give you a nice visual over any problem areas, identify personal patterns, and make viable changes for yourself.*

staying away for good

When you truly decide to walk away from the narcissist, staying away for good is often the hardest part. It's not just about leaving the person; it's also about leaving behind the emotional bonds, the shared history, and mostly the illusions of what you thought the relationship could be like in the future. Healing requires your full, long-term commitment, massive amounts of self-awareness, and a lot of willpower. It's not an easy path, but it's a worthwhile one.

missing your abuser

During your healing journey, you will encounter some very hard moments. It's natural to find yourself missing your abuser, even months or years later, even when you know the relationship was toxic and harmful. This doesn't make you weak, and it doesn't mean you're failing in your growth. Missing them is a reflection of the love you gave, the hopes you had, and the dreams you built around them. It's a sign of your humanity, your empathy, and your ability to love someone—not a sign that you should go back. You might long for the good moments, the rare times they made you feel seen, loved, or safe. But remember, those moments were not the whole story. Missing your abuser is a process of grieving what you thought it could be, not what it truly was.

It's important to understand that missing someone isn't the same as needing them. You can miss the comfort of familiarity, the shared memories, or the illusion of love they created while still knowing deep down that your decision to leave was the right one. This tug-of-war between your heart and mind is part of healing; it's messy and painful, but it's also where transformation begins. There will be difficult situations where you feel discouraged or triggered. Let yourself feel the sadness without judgment; it's a natural part of the grieving process. Cry if you need to. Curl into a ball and forget the world, even weeks and months after the fact. Write it out. Talk about it with someone you trust. But don't mistake the pain of missing them for a sign that you should reach out or go back.

Instead, take these moments of longing as opportunities to strengthen your resolve. Reflect on what you deserve: love without conditions, kindness without manipulation, and a life where your happiness isn't contingent on someone else's control. Use this time to redirect that longing back to yourself. What are you truly craving in those moments? Is it safety, love, or validation? These are things you can—and will—provide for yourself as you continue to heal. Remember, missing them doesn't mean you're losing; it means you're learning to let go. Each time you face this feeling and move through it, you are another step closer to the freedom and peace you deserve.

Last but not least, you will meet many new, inspiring people and might feel the urge to run away from them immediately, especially if it feels like another sacred connection or very strong chemistry. Do not run away, but embrace these connections in a smart way by cross-checking everything you have learned. Instead of avoiding these moments, put in the work so you can enjoy your life again to the fullest!

further reminders to help you stay free

It's understandable you may not yet trust your own judgment 100 percent. To ensure you don't fall for another narcissist, follow these suggestions.

- No contact with your ex, no matter what.

- Reread this book as many times as you wish. Stick to it as your little "bible of staying healthy." Do not deviate from your path.

- Get into a routine and try not to deviate until you feel 100 percent again.

- Put your mental health first, no matter what.

- Get *My Toxic Breakup—A Guided Journal* and fill it out for thirty-five days. Reread all the work you put in, as many times as you need to.

- Make sure you can recognize the twenty-four toxic traits, or watch my video at https://stan.store/alinakastner/p/spot-toxicity-now.

- Visit my Healing Your Heart series at https://stan.store/alinakastner/p/begin -your-healing-journey.

- When you meet someone, go back to the section on dating and cross-check the questions and lists. Give it some time (at least six months), and check for consistency before making any decisions to take this relationship anywhere more committed. If the known red flags pop up, withdraw as quickly as you can.

- Try healthy relationship hypnosis with Claudia Schwinghammer. Claudia and I work together in helping people find healthy relationships after abuse. Through her specialized hypnosis therapy, she programs a client's subconscious to never react to a narcissist again. She will do a one-off hypnosis session with my clients once they are ready to move on to new relationships and provide them with a twenty-one-day audio to listen to afterward. Her success rate with my clients so far is above 93 percent, and people are truly enjoying their love life after working with her. She does her work online, so you can access her help from all over the world, and she speaks perfect English. Find her when you are ready to date again at https://mental-health.wien/en.

Follow my channels:

- Instagram: @dr.alinakastner
- TikTok: @dr.alinakastner
- Website: www.alinakastner.com

Find all my services, appointments, workshops, podcasts, and free playlists at @stan.store/alinakastner.

Follow these people (or five people of your choosing) on Instagram for an extra sprinkle of life and narc wisdom and get into all they have to offer (podcasts, books, daily meditations, and more).

- @_synful_
- @jillianturecki
- @gabormatemd
- @rl_soul
- @manifestelle

If you are committed to your goal of staying narc-free and following all the advice in this book, you will see that your efforts will 100 percent pay off. You will flourish and feel much better in time, I promise you. All you need to do is stay consistent and be patient. Once the narc is completely out of your life and you no longer tolerate toxicity, they can no longer contaminate you with their poison. You will begin to regain strength day by day, as they no longer have the power to weaken you.

chapter 12

love letters

*"Almost everything will work again if you unplug
it for a few minutes, including you"*

—Anne Lamott

T o end this book, I'd love your assistance. I want you to help create a beautiful ending to the first part of our journey together—and a beautiful beginning to your newly paved path. This will happen in three ways: receiving love from those closest to you, from your own heart, and from mine.

love letters to you, from loved ones

Ask at least three trusted friends or loving family members to write you a love letter. Yes—a real, heartfelt letter just for you. Explain your situation and let them know how much it would mean to you if you received a few soul-nourishing messages from them. Ask them to send their letters by mail over the next few months. Ideally, they'll arrive spaced out: one now, another in a month, the next a month after that, so you have something uplifting to open every so often. This external perspective can reinforce your beautifully growing self-worth and remind you of your strong support network in times of doubt!

a love letter to yourself

Next, I want you to send some love your own way. For this, grab a beautiful piece of paper and your favorite pen—and just trust me. I want you to write yourself a love letter. Make it kind, tender, and compassionate. Let it be the most meaningful love letter you've ever received.

Imagine you are writing to someone you deeply cherish—someone who has fought battles they never deserved to fight yet got through them with all their courage and resilience and are now stronger than ever. Now realize that this cherished person is you! Settle into a space where you feel calm and safe. Let your shoulders drop, take a deep breath, and feel the weight of the journey you've survived lift, if only for a moment. This is your time, your moment to honor yourself and your heartbreak.

Remind yourself of all the battles you've faced and acknowledge how much strength and dedication it took for you to get through it and finally step away from the toxic grip of the narcissist. Be as proud of yourself as I am of you, and feel the words "I deserve better" while you write. Write about your growth, the moments of clarity, the lessons you have learned, and the small but mighty victories along the way. Let yourself be proud and full of love and gratefulness for how far you have come. Thank yourself for not giving up at any point in time and for protecting the tender parts of your soul even when they felt fragile and exposed. Write with gratitude for the strength that carried you through your darkest days and the light that now begins to shine inside you, brighter with each passing moment as you move toward healing your heart fully.

As you write, allow love to flow freely—love for the person you've been, the person you are, and the person you are becoming. Let forgiveness find its way into your words, not just for others but also for yourself, for the moments when you didn't know what you know now. I am sending you all my love while you write this most important love letter of your life. Let your words be a reminder that you are a survivor, a thriver, and above all, a deeply deserving human being. When you finish, take a moment to reread what you've written. Feel the love you've poured into those words and know that it is yours, always. If you feel overwhelmed about where to start, perhaps you can draw a little inspiration from these prompts:

Dear Me,

- I am writing this letter to you, because _____
- I am in awe of you for _____
- I love you because _____
- I don't tell you this enough, but _____
- Thank you for _____
- You have shown me _____
- I am so proud of you for _____
- You are so powerful because _____
- I know you are enough because _____
- I celebrate you for _____
- You inspire me because _____
- I admire the way you _____
- You have taught me that _____
- I want to remind you that _____
- I see your strength when _____
- You amaze me with your ability to _____
- I feel so grateful for the way you _____
- You have every right to _____
- I honor the part of you that _____
- You are healing beautifully by _____
- You have the courage to _____
- I cherish the moments when you _____
- You are radiant because _____
- You are becoming someone who _____
- I see how far you've come from _____
- I believe in your ability to _____
- You deserve _____
- I will make sure you know _____
- I forgive you for _____
- I promise to _____

With all my love, *Me*

my love letter to you

My Dear One,

We are at the end of our shared journey through this book, though it does not have to be the end of our journey together. Find me on my socials, keep in touch, and please reach out to let me know how this book helped you. I am so very proud of you for making it to this point and grateful that you stuck with me through these final pages. I would feel deeply honored to be tagged in a post of this book once you hold it in your hands and would repost with joy.

I want you to pause for a moment here and look back. Look at all the pages you read, all the check-ins you did, all the reflection you did, all the advice you took, and all the wisdom you learned from the many great teachers you have met in real life, in digital life, or in this book. It takes so much strength to face the aftermath of abuse, and you are taking the steps toward building a new life for yourself.

Your journey does not end here, and it does not end with this book. Each day forward is your chance to finally live the life you have wanted for yourself and honor all the work you've already done! This next chapter of your life is so powerful—full of love and clarity. There is absolutely no more space for anyone who doesn't truly see your worth, as you see it now! I see it too. I know exactly how strong you are. Put your faith in the process, and remember your future is yours alone. Go out there and live it fully and freely.

Don't ever forget it: You are worthy, whole, and capable of creating a beautiful, fulfilling life. This is only the beginning of the rest of your journey.

With all my love and healing energy,

Alina

resources

further reading

Kastner, Alina. *My Toxic Breakup—A Guided Journal*. Self-Published, Amazon Digital Services, 2024.

"24 Toxic Traits" Video: https://stan.store/alinakastner/p/spot-toxicity-now

Healing Your Heart series: https://stan.store/alinakastner/p/begin-your-healing-journey.

Dechaos.org provides education on narcissism and offers narcissistic survivors the opportunity to share their personal stories. They host in-person events.

Narcissisticman.com is a website created for narcissistic abuse survivors and gives them the opportunity to join online groups.

bibliography

American Psychiatric Association. *Diagnostic and Statistical Manual of Mental Disorders*, Text Revision DSM-5-TR. 5th ed. Arlington, VA: American Psychiatric Publishing, 2022.

Arabi, Shahida. *Becoming the Narcissist's Nightmare: How to Devalue and Discard the Narcissist While Supplying Yourself*. Scottsdale, AZ: SCW Archer Publishing, 2017.

Behary, Wendy. *Disarming the Narcissist: Surviving and Thriving with the Self-Absorbed*. 3rd ed. Oakland, CA: New Harbinger Publications, 2021

Bennice, Jennifer A, et al. "The Relative Effects of Intimate Partner Physical and Sexual Violence on Post-Traumatic Stress Disorder Symptomatology." *Violence and Victims* 18, no. 1 (2003): 87–94. https://doi.org/10.1891/vivi.2003.18.1.87.

Brach, Tara. *Radical Acceptance: Embracing Your Life with the Heart of a Buddha*. New York: Bantam Books, 2003.

Campbell, W. Keith. "Narcissism and Romantic Attraction." *Journal of Personality and Social Psychology* 77, no. 6 (1999): 1254–70. https://doi.org/10.1037/0022-3514.77.6.1254.

Carlson, Jon, Katherine Helm, and Len Sperry. *The Disordered Couple*. 2nd ed. New York: Routledge, 2017.

Fleischman, Diana. "Sex as Bonding Mechanisms." In *Encyclopedia of Evolutionary Psychological Science*, edited by Todd K. Shackelford, Viviana A. Weekes-Shackelford, 7062–63. Chams, Switzerland: Springer, 2021. https://doi.org/10.1007/978-3-319-19650-3_1717.

Gottman, J. M., and N. Silver. *The Seven Principles for Making Marriage Work: A Practical Guide from the Country's Foremost Relationship Expert*. New York: Harmony Books, 2015.

Grand, David. "Brainspotting: A New Brain-Based Psychotherapy Approach." *Trauma & Gewalt* 5, no. 3 (2011): 276.

Herman, Judith Lewis. "Complex PTSD: A Syndrome in Survivors of Prolonged and Repeated Trauma." *Journal of Traumatic Stress* 5, no. 3 (1992): 377–91. https://doi.org/10.1002/jts.2490050305.

Hill, Jess. *See What You Made Me Do: The Dangers of Domestic Abuse That We Ignore, Explain Away, or Refuse to See*. Naperville, IL: Sourcebooks, 2020.

Horvath, Adam O., and B. Diane Symonds. "Relation Between Working Alliance and Outcome in Psychotherapy: A Meta-Analysis." *Journal of Counseling Psychology* 38, no. 2 (1991): 139–49. https://doi.org/10.1037/0022-0167.38.2.139.

Howard, Vickie. "Recognizing Narcissistic Abuse and the Implications for Mental Health Nursing Practice." *Issues in Mental Health Nursing* 40, no. 8 (2019): 644–54. https://doi.org/10.1080/01612840.2019.1590485.

Kabat-Zinn, Jon. "An Outpatient Program in Behavioral Medicine for Chronic Pain Patients Based on the Practice of Mindfulness Meditation: Theoretical Considerations and Preliminary Results." *General Hospital Psychiatry* 4, no. 1 (1982): 33–47. https://doi.org/10.1016/0163-8343(82)90026-3.

Kabat-Zinn, Jon. *Full Catastrophe Living: Using the Wisdom of Your Body and Mind to Face Stress, Pain, and Illness*. Rev. ed. New York: Bantam, 2013.

Kastner-Bosek, Alina, et al. "Addicted to Self-Esteem: Understanding the Neurochemistry of Narcissism by Using Cocaine as a Pharmacological Model." *Journal of Experimental Psychopathology* 12, no. 3 (2021): 204380872110443. https://doi.org/10.1177/20438087211044362.

Kernberg, Otto F. *Borderline Conditions and Pathological Narcissism*. New York: Jason Aronson, 1995.

Kübler-Ross, Elisabeth. *On Death and Dying*. New York: Macmillan, 1969.

Leventhal, Allan M. "Sadness, Depression, and Avoidance Behavior." *Behavior Modification* 32, no. 6 (2008): 759–79. https://doi.org/10.1177/0145445508317167.

MacKenzie, Jackson. *Psychopath Free: Recovering from Emotionally Abusive Relationships with Narcissists, Sociopaths, and Other Toxic People*. New York: Berkley Books, 2015.

Määttä, Marju, Satu Uusiautti, and Kaarina Määttä. "An Intimate Relationship in the Shadow of Narcissism: What Is It Like to Live with a Narcissistic Spouse?" *International Journal of Research Studies in Psychology* 1, no. 1 (2012): 28–42. https://doi.org/10.5861/ijrsp.2012.v1i1.28.

O'Haire, Marguerite E., Noemie A. Gurin, and Alison C. Kirkham. "Animal-Assisted Intervention for Trauma: A Systematic Literature Review." *Frontiers in Psychology* 6 (2015): 1121. https://doi.org/10.3389/fpsyg.2015.01121.

Reid, Joan, et al. "Trauma Bonding and Interpersonal Violence." *Psychology of Trauma* 2013.

Reviere, S. et al. "Intimate Partner Abuse and Suicide." *Journal of Family Violence* 22 (2007).

Tedeschi, Philip, Aubrey H. Fine, and Jana I. Helgeson. "Assistance Animals." *In Handbook on Animal-Assisted Therapy: Foundations and Guidelines for Animal-Assisted Interventions*, edited by Aubrey H. Fine, 421–38. San Diego, CA: Academic Press, 2010. https://doi.org/10.1016/b978-0-12-381453-1.10020-0.

Thomas, Shannon. *Healing from Hidden Abuse: A Journey Through the Stages of Recovery from Psychological Abuse*. MAST Publishing House, 2016.

Tortoriello, Gregory K. "Do Narcissists Try to Make Romantic Partners Jealous on Purpose?" *Personality and Individual Differences* 114 (2017): 10–15. https://doi.org/10.1016/j.paid.2017.03.052.

acknowledgments

First and foremost, I want to thank my son, Maximilian, for showing me what it truly means to love. To quote X Ambassadors, "I've been living a half life, my whole life, till I loved you." I will always try my best to help you be true to yourself and be someone who treats others with a genuine understanding of love. You are my greatest inspiration for this book and my hope for a kinder world.

To Matthäus, a loving partner in crime, thank you for gifting me Max and always being there for us. I love you from the bottom of my heart.

To my other kiddos—Amari, Bonnie, Lolita, Medea, Soñada, and Tsunami—who have been there for years, always having my back, always full of love, and always saying so much without saying a word. You have helped me and many of my clients heal in so many ways, and I cannot thank you enough.

To C., Ma., and Mo., thank you for being the boys who forced me to grow up quicker than I should have had to. You hurt me badly, perhaps without malicious intent, but you taught me the necessity of self-love. And to B., my biggest teacher of all, who hurt me so deeply with his narcissism that I felt a calling to protect others from this kind of pain by writing this book. Thank you for this bittersweet motivation.

To Jill, my publishing momma, the true founder of this book's vision. Thank you for all your guidance on the how-tos of creating a book from scratch. Thank you for believing in me and our baby, holding me up and having my back when time schedules rushed and things felt very stressful.

To Karen, my development editor, thank you for guiding me through every stage of shaping this book. Your patience really helped me relax, and your fantastic insights and commitment helped shape this raw stone into a diamond!

To Emily, my copy editor, thank you for your keen eye for detail. Your meticulous editing and insightful suggestions have truly elevated this book.

To Ismita, my marketing manager, a big thank-you for your calming presence and incredible energy. You made the process so much smoother and helped keep me grounded.

To Kate, whose talent brought this book's design to life. Your keen eye for detail made all the difference, and I am incredibly grateful for your invaluable support.

To my mom, who gave me the strength to trust myself and be independent, even when life got hard. Thank you for always being there in ways big and small, shaping the woman I am today.

To my dad, who taught me what it means to never argue for your limitations. You taught me the power of radical acceptance and brought me closer to the wisdom of Krishnamurti, forever reminding me that "the ability to observe without evaluating is the highest form of intelligence."

To my Aunt Stella, my big cheerleader, your support and guidance have been a constant light and a source of strength for me. To Reini and Eris, for supporting her with all their hearts.

To my sisters: L., the first love of my life, thank you for showing me the meaning of healing after heartbreak. Losing the relationship we once shared was the hardest lesson ever, but I am grateful for every piece of growth that pain has given me. N., thank you for showing me how to be an absolute fighter and how to cheat death and get away with it. And thank you, R., for giving me the greatest gift anyone has ever given me—a gift so transformative, I wouldn't be here without it.

To my best friends—Alona, Ana, Britta, Carlos, Claudia, Gelena, Jenny, Josh, Kate, Kathi, Lara, Lisa, Maria, Nina, Patrizia, Ruedilyn, Sean, Susi, and Vici—thank you for reminding me that friends are the family you choose. Sharing our sob stories (especially those involving narcs!) the past years inspired this book in many ways, and I am endlessly thankful. Our shared journeys have reminded me that even in the hardest times, I am never alone, and there is always humor, hugs, and a love that only true friends can provide.

To Nathalie and Rimma, for cleansing my spirit, connecting me with higher grounds and making sure that life can grow inside of me. This book is part of that life's creation.

To all my dear clients and followers, thank you for your courage and openness in allowing me into your lives. You shared your deepest truths, your struggles, and your moments of resilience with me, trusting me to be a part of your healing journey. Each session, each story, has been a privilege and a reminder of the strength that lies in vulnerability. This has inspired me deeply and shaped every chapter of this book. I am endlessly grateful for the honor of walking alongside you in your path to healing.

To the clients that have let me share your very personal stories in this book: Your bravery to confront the past so openly and share it with the world is inspiring. It takes more than courage to do this, and I am endlessly grateful for your contribution. I believe it has made this book come to life and will help all my readers understand the essence of abuse and the essence of healing much better.

And finally, to all of you who are holding this book in your hands, all my dear readers. Thank you for trusting me with your journey. I hope this book brings you healing, hope, and the strength to keep moving forward, narcissist-free!

Last but not least: to me, myself, and I—who chose courage over fear every time. You might be my biggest role model going forward.

With all my heart, *Alina*

about the author

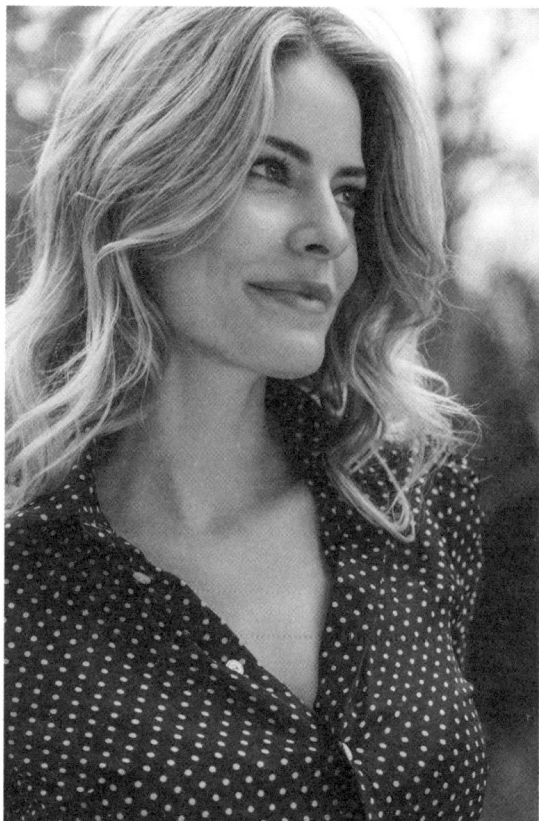

©LUISE REICHERT

Dr. Alina Kastner is a systemic family therapist specializing in narcissism, emotional abuse, and sex therapy. Blending her clinical expertise with research and compassion, she is dedicated to helping clients heal and rebuild their lives. Based in Austria with her son, dog, and horses, Alina shares practical advice and insights on Instagram, TikTok, and YouTube (@dr.alinakastner). *Break Up with Narcissism: How to Break Free and Stay Free* is her debut book, a powerful guide to breaking free from the grip of narcissistic abuse. Learn more at www.alinakastner.com.

index

Quarto.com

© 2026 Quarto Publishing
Text © 2026 Alina Kastner

First Published in 2026 by Fair Winds Press, an imprint of The Quarto Group,
100 Cummings Center, Suite 265-D, Beverly, MA 01915, USA.
T (978) 282-9590 F (978) 283-2742

EEA Representation, WTS Tax d.o.o.,
Žanova ulica 3, 4000 Kranj, Slovenia.
www.wts-tax.si

Fair Winds Press titles are also available at discount for retail, wholesale, promotional, and bulk purchase.
For details, contact the Special Sales Manager by email at specialsales@quarto.com or by mail at The
Quarto Group, Attn: Special Sales Manager, 100 Cummings Center, Suite 265-D, Beverly, MA 01915, USA.

30 29 28 27 26   1 2 3 4 5

ISBN: 978-0-7603-9523-3

Digital edition published in 2026
eISBN: 978-0-7603-9524-0

Library of Congress Cataloging-in-Publication Data available

Cover Design: Tanya Jacobson
Interior Design: tabula rasa graphic design

Printed in Malaysia

The information in this book is for educational purposes only. It is not intended to replace the advice of a
physician or medical practitioner. The publisher is not responsible for any loss, damage, or consequences
arising from the use of this publication.